Sirtfood Diet

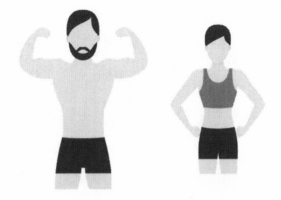

by Julia Meadows

About the Author

Julia Meadows is a senior coach at Mindset Mastership, a life coaching business based in London, England.

Mindset Mastership teaches clients how human behavior really works. Through our teaching, we have helped clients worldwide gain a better advantage, to develop themselves and achieve more from life.

For further details, see:

MindsetMastership.com

Want free goodies?

Email us at:

mindsetmastership@gmail.com

Find us on Instagram!

@MindsetMastership

The SirtFood Diet

Discover the international diet sensation—As used by *Adele*, heavyweight champion *David Haye*, and *Pippa Middleton*

— this diet will help you lose weight from fat and not muscle AND ensure you look, feel better and energised days while eating all the foods you love.

Table of Contents

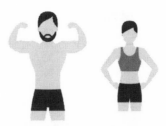

Introduction:

The SirtFood Diet

Discover the groundbreaking international diet sensation—As used by singer Adele, heavyweight champion David Haye, and royalty Pippa Middleton.

This diet can help you lose weight and burn fat, maintain muscle AND ensure you look and feel better, maintaining energized days while eating all the foods you love.

Imagine yourself with a slimmer waist, leaner body, more muscle and less fat? Then the Sirtfood diet is for you!

In this Sirtfood diet cookbook you will discover the secrets to how celebrities lose weight, burn fat or get lean by activating your "skinny gene". You will also get a stress-free step-by-step plan with easy to cook healthy preps & delicious recipe ideas, all included!

In this book we reveal:

- **A complete understanding of the SirtFood Diet and how it works**
- Step-by-step cooking and recipes with instructions
- **Complete cheatsheet of Sirtfoods that work**
- How to build muscle or get leaner
- **How to lose weight & burn fat**
- How to maintain a healthy lifestyle

The Sirtfood diet will help you lose 7 pounds in 7 days.

This book also includes a list of Sirtfoods that also help to reduce inflammation which also includes anti-aging properties.

Do something to change the way you feel about yourself.

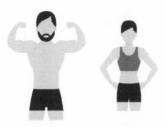

Chapter 1:
The Science of Sirtuins

The sirtfood diet is based on research on SIRTs or sirtuins. These are a group of seven proteins found in the human body that regulate functions like metabolism as well as inflammation and lifespan. The sirtfood diet works on the assumption that certain plant compounds may be able to increase the level of these proteins. These plants are dubbed "sirtfoods".

A combination of sirtfoods along with calorie restriction could trigger the body to produce higher levels of sirtuins, leading to rapid weight loss, while maintaining muscle mass.

OF MICE AND MEN

In recent times, sirtuins have, unsurprisingly, become the focus of extensive scientific investigation. The first sirtuin was detected in yeast back in 1984, but research really began over the span of the next 30 years when it was realized that sirtuin stimulation enhances lifespan, first in yeast then all the way to mice.

Why the thrill? Because from yeast to humans and everything else in between, the basic values of cell metabolism are remarkably similar. If you can control anything as small as a burgeoning yeast to see a gain and replicate it in a higher species like mice, there is hope for the same advantages in humans.

AN APPETITE FOR FASTING?

This brings us to fasting. Continuously, a lifetime reduction of food consumption has been found to increase the lifespan of lower species and mammals. This awesome finding is the foundation for the practice of caloric restriction among certain people, where regularly calorie intake is decreased by around twenty to thirty percent. Such fasting helped popularize the offshoot, irregular fasting, that has become an effective weight-loss solution, partly inspired by the likes of the 5:2 or Fast Diet. While we're still waiting for evidence of an increased lifetime for human beings from these procedures, there's evidence of advantages to what we might call the "health period" where chronic disease drops and fat falls ebb.

But let's be truthful, no matter how great the advantages, dieting week in and week out is an exhausting business that many of us don't want to sign up for. Even when we do, most of us are not prepared to adhere to such rigor. Nevertheless there are disadvantages to fasting, particularly if we follow it for a long time. We listed in the intro the adverse effects of hunger, tiredness, weakness, muscular failure and slowing of the metabolic rate. But continuing fasting schemes could also put us at risk of food insecurity, impacting our health due to the reduction of fats nutrients. Fasting systems are often entirely inadequate for vast numbers of the population such as infants, women during gestation, and most likely older people. Although fasting obviously has proven advantages, it's not the silver bullet we 'd want. Is the way Nature meant to make us thin, fit, and active? There's obviously another good way out there.

Our discovery came when we learned that our old sirtuin genes were enabled by mediating the substantial advantages of caloric restriction and abstinence. Thinking of sirtuins as the defenders at the intersection of energy status and immortality may be beneficial to fully understand this. What they do is react to stress and strain.

When energy is in limited supply, there is a rise in tension in our cells from the calorie limit. The sirtuins detected this and then turn on and transmit a series of potent signals that dramatically altered cell behavior. Sirtuins start increasing our metabolism and our muscular productivity, switch on fat loss, reduce pain and fix cell damage. Sirtuins, in turn, make us fit and healthy, slimmer, and safer.

There are 7 distinct sirtuins in humans (SIRT1 to SIRT7). Of these, the single most significant associated with energy equilibrium are SIRT1 and SIRT3. Although SIRT1 is present in the body, SIRT3 is located mainly in the mitochondria—the cells' energy-main house. Their stimulation next to each other affords us the many advantages we are hoping to achieve.

A ZEAL FOR EXERCISE?

It isn't just caloric limitation and fasting that trigger sirtuins; exercise also does. As in fasting, sirtuins organize the profound advantages of a workout. Yet while we are urged to participate in a routine of physical activity for its myriad of advantages, it is not the mechanism by which we are expected to concentrate our attention on weight-loss. Evidence indicates that the human body has developed ways of adapting spontaneously and that the energy and power we generate while exercising ensure for fitness to be a successful weight-loss strategy requires the devotion of lots of time and effort. Grueling fitness regimens as the way evolution designed us to sustain a healthier weight seems much more questionable in the face of studies now showing that exercising too much may be dangerous and undermine our immune systems, damage the heart, and lead to early mortality.

ENTER SIRTFOODS

So far, we realize that the key to activating our sirtuin genes is wanting to lose some weight and be healthful. Fasting and meditation have been the 2 main ways of doing that up to now. Unfortunately, the positives for good weight loss come with disadvantages; but for most of us, this is clearly inconsistent with how we lead 21st century lives. Luckily, there is a recent ground-breaking way to activate our sirtuin genes in the most effective manner possible: sirtfood. As we will soon discover, these are the miracle foods especially abundant in unique plant natural chemicals, which have the capacity to converse with our sirtuin genes and turn them on. In fact, they imitate the impact of abstinence and workout and in doing so offer incredible advantages of weight loss, muscle strengthening, and better health that were formerly unachievable.

SUMMARY

- We each have an ancestral gene group, called sirtuins.
- Primary metabolic controllers are sirtuins that regulate our capacity to lose fat and remain alive.
- Sirtuins serve as energy detectors in our cells and are triggered when energy deficits are observed.
- Fasting and workout both stimulate our sirtuin genes but may be difficult to adhere to and even have disadvantages.
- Our sirtuin genes are being programmed in a new innovative way: sirtfoods.
- You can counteract the action of fasting and workout by eating a diet rich in sirtfoods and accomplish the body you desire.

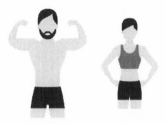

Chapter 2:
Sirtfoods Explained

WHAT ARE SIRTS?

SIRTs, or sirtuins, are a group of enzymes that control key biological cell growth reactions. Owing to their ability to improve fat loss, super increasing your activity levels and perhaps even prolonging your life, their discovery has created tremendous anticipation.

The very first SIRT was identified in yeast cells and assigned the SIR2 (Silent Information Regulator 2) protein, an unexceptional name. SIRTs or sirtuins are related proteins eventually discovered in human cells. 7 human SIRT proteins have been found already and have been titled SIRT1 to SIRT7.

WHAT DO SIRTS DO?

Sirtuin proteins are enzymes that play a critical part in how cells adapt to meals, exercise as well as other lifestyle influences. SIRTs operate with the cells, fine-tuning their output so that each cell works more effectively. They achieve this by modifying the chemical composition of different proteins and fatty acids present in the cell nuclei, cell liquid (cytoplasm) and energy-producing cell components (mitochondria).

This specific alteration inside the nucleus (the most important of which is a synthetic snip known as diacylation) leads to the activation or inhibition of cell genes involved. Such gene modifications, combined, allow the cells to:

- Turbocharge and generate cellular capacity
- Boost reducing fat
- Facilitate favorable weight loss
- Trigger channels for cell protection to reduce inflammation
- Repair DNA harmed
- Regrow worn out components of cells (organelles)
- Lengthen the cell viability during stressful periods due to factors such as lack of oxygen, disease, or pathogen build-up

- Place new synaptic connections within the brain to facilitate memory development, preservation, and recovery.

Each sirtuin protein is focused to function inside of particular parts of each cell.

SIRT1, SIRT6, and SIRT7 are found primarily in the cell nucleus and are involved in the regulation of how genes are managed to switch on and off in reply to certain stimuli – including all those genes responsible for the SIRT proteins themselves. SIRT7 mostly focuses inside the nuclear membrane in an area known as the nucleolus, where the protein-making apparatus of the cell is controlled.

SIRT2 is predominantly found in cell plasma (cytoplasm) where it controls cellular metabolism and also cell regeneration and DNA repair associated anti-aging activities.

SIRT3, SIRT4, and SIRT5 are found primarily inside the mitochondria – the relatively small ever-ready devices that produce energy in each cell. SIRT3 is intimately correlated with the process of aging and long life while SIRT4 has a particular insulin sensitivity-related action.

FOOD SAFETY MISTAKES

1. Transporting groceries from the store to home

One basic principle is to keep foods frozen or refrigerated at all times. Even at a slow pace, microbes grow rapidly in food once they start to warm up.

If it takes you more than 30 minutes to get to your home from the grocery store, plan ahead and keep a cooler inside your car with an ice pack! Ideally stop at the grocery store as the last part of your food trip.

If you're not using a cooler but go straight home, keep the perishable food in front of your car where there is air conditioning and it's cooler. Keep in mind that perishables can only be kept in a cooler for around two hours till microbes start to develop.

2. Properly reheating leftovers

Leftover food is always a great option, especially if you're crunched for time, but did you know that not properly heating leftovers is a major cause of foodborne disease?

First and foremost: Ensure that the leftovers are refrigerated properly when putting them away. Many people assume that leftovers need to be cooled first, but that actually increases microbe development, so get them in the fridge asap (at least within 2 hours).

Second: Cook your food to at least 165 degrees F or until the food is steaming (if you are super vigilant you can use a food thermometer to double check). Using microwaves to heat up leftovers is very common, although not always consistent with heating food all the way through, so double check that your entire item is hot before consuming.

3. Cross contamination

Cross contamination is currently the leading cause of foodborne disease. Think BBQ meats put back in same dish in which they were marinated. It's also one of the easiest food safety errors to fix with a little attention.

As long as you separate ready-to-eat foods and clean utensils from materials that may have come into contact with raw meats, you're more likely to be in the clear. Do not hesitate to scrub your cutting boards! (Wash them in wet, soapy water and if you really want to keep them clean, spritz or rinse them with white vinegar. You can place plastic boards in a dishwasher to sanitize them.

These safety measures are significant since raw meat bacteria are extremely easy to transfer.

4. Thawing frozen foods

Everybody has learned a way to thaw frozen foods, but actually there was a right or wrong way to do it ... and most of us are messing it up.

Actually, only 62 percent of people thaw their frozen foods correctly. Frozen foods must be defrosted NOT on the countertop because the food can attain a temperature of between 40-140 degrees F which is "the danger zone" for food safety experts. This maximum temperature is where pathogens multiply the most rapidly. Even if you don't think this is risky, it is.

The finest (and safest) way to thaw frozen food is in your refrigerator. This helps the frozen item to thaw gradually without going into "the danger zone." if that isn't possible and you fail to thaw your steak for dinner, you can defrost any frozen food in a big bowl of cool water (just make sure it's in an airtight box or plastic bag. And don't forget it overnight on the counter!.

5. Not washing your Hands (or not washing them properly)

This one looks simple but could very easily get you sick. Wash your hands after handling raw poultry, meat, fish, or eggs. Which means BEFORE you touch anything. Use tongs or even a kitchen mitt, when your hands are not well cleaned, because pathogens expand to EVERYTHING you contact. And no, putting your hands under water doesn't count.

To reduce pathogen spread you should wash your hands with soap and warm water. Most people don't wash their hands as thoroughly (or as frequently) as they should. A thumb rule is to wash your hands for as long as it takes to recite the ABC's. This may sound a little (or very) dumb, but it guarantees you don't spread bacteria in your kitchen.

6. Using a raw meat marinade on cooked meat

The last thing you want to think about when relaxing at a BBQ is food poisoning. While marinating your meat before cooking is a good practice, you should NOT use a marinade with which raw meat has come into contact. Go for a fresh batch as a sauce or boil it first to destroy any nasty pathogens.

7. Not replacing (or sanitizing) sponges and dishrags

Cross-contamination is super normal as discussed above, but have you ever thought about all the bacteria harboring in your sponge and dish rags?

Like cutting boards, sponges and dishrags are porous which make them a breeding ground for pathogens and germs. It is best to sanitize sponges every other day to avoid this (you can soak them in white vinegar, run them through the dishwasher, or nuke them in the microwave (when wet!) for 60 seconds on "high" and sometimes just replace them.

And please don't use the dishwashing sponges to wipe down your counters! That commits mistake #3!

Make it a routine to wash your kitchen towels 2-3x a week (ideally in HOT water) or more frequently as needed. This will make sure that pathogens don't spread around your kitchen.

8. Washing poultry before preparing

Raw poultry is one of the food products most often polluted. Perhaps that's why some people get used to "cleaning" it by rinsing it in the sink before cooking, but it's currently been shown to expand bacteria around the kitchen. Chicken water droplets (even the small ones you can't see) are a possible source of contamination.

In particular, any surface it touches should be disinfected when preparing poultry - or any meat for that matter. But cleaning meat increases the region that needs disinfection. Unfortunately, we are not superhuman, so when washed, we cannot see every place the poultry touches.

If food safety is essential to you, it is better not to wash the poultry before preparing it and instead ensure that you cook it at the proper temperature to kill any pathogens (165 degrees F).

9. Assuming raw vegetables are safe

This could be the biggest misconception people have concerning food safety. Many of us believe we can only get sick from raw meat but do you know that salmonella can be harbored in a cantaloupe's rind? Or that leafy greens often become contaminated with E. coli?

Fresh produce accounts for almost half of food-borne illnesses, so in reality it is very important to properly prepare and store produce. Ensure that perishable products are kept in a refrigerator in a crisper drawer and are not handled with dirty hands. Rinse your produce before eating (use a diluted mixture of vinegar-water to help reduce surface bacteria). Buying local farmers' produce decreases the risk of food poisoning, as many of the products responsible for major outbreaks have been related to contamination in giant processing plants.

10. Separation of food in the fridge

Most people put food anywhere they can find room in their refrigerator, but in reality, there is a proper way to place food to avoid contamination.

So, what's the best order?

Raw meat must be placed on the fridge's absolute bottom shelf. This is because meat packets are likely to spill liquid, creating a nightmare of contamination if placed on the top shelf. (Still better, put meat in a bag or on a plate to catch any leaks.) Also, perishable products should be kept in the refrigerator's bottom drawers to remove them from any possible contamination from other contents. Keep clean those veggie drawers!

PROS AND CONS:

Pros:

- The "sirt foods" are expected to activate your body's sirtuin, a form of protein that helps to protect your cells from dying and developing diseases while controlling metabolism.
- It is based on a sample of 40 gym-goers who each lost 7 lbs. in a week without losing muscle mass.
- You may regularly have small doses of dark chocolate and wine without feeling guilty!
- It includes generally safe, nutritious foods such as buckwheat, blueberries, walnuts, and green tea
- It is basically designed to keep you safe for life and to delay the aging process

Cons:

- There is a calorie limit for the first week that would no doubt cause most people to lose weight, regardless of what foods they eat. This means that the participants may be losing weight due to the calorie restriction itself. For the first three days you only eat 1,000 calories a day, and then the next four days 1,500 calories per day.

- Restricting your calorie intake drastically can be dangerous if your body isn't used to it and you can feel lethargic.
- There is not enough evidence that its promises, especially the acceleration metabolism, are being followed through. A 40-person study is not large enough to say it will certainly work as a sustainable way to lose weight.
- Only foods such as sirt juices, rocket, soy, green tea and walnuts can be on the sirt food list.

As a consequence of the above, less focus is put on incorporating a variety of foods into your diet so you can look and feel fantastic. Eating a rainbow of fruits and vegetables every day, for example, means you get a range of vitamins and minerals in your meals.

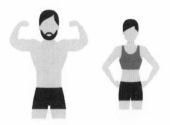

Chapter 3:
Best Sirtfoods

FOOD NAMED

Now that you know enough about sirtfoods, why they're so good and what it takes to build a successful diet that will produce lifelong results, it's time to get started. Now is the best time to get started with each of the top twenty sirtfoods that will shortly become the basics of your daily diet.

Arugula

Clearly, Arugula (also known as rocket, rucola, rugula, and roquette) has a vivid history in American food culture. A musky green salad leaf with a prominent peppery flavor, it soon advanced from its humble beginnings as the foundation of many Mediterranean farm dishes to become an emblem of food snobbery in many countries, thus contributing to the popularization of the word arugulance!

However long before it became a salad leaf in a battle of dominance, arugula became valued for its healing qualities by the ancient Greeks and Romans. Frequently used as a diuretic and nutritional aid, it earned its true renown for possessing strong aphrodisiac powers, so much so that arugula production was prohibited in Middle Ages monasteries. It is also famous for arousing the sexual appetite of drowsy men.

However, what really excites us about arugula is the booming quantities of the sirtuin-activating kaempferol and quercetin nutrients. A mixture of kaempferol and quercetin is being studied as a topical product in addition to its existing sirtuin-activating effects, as together they promote collagen production in the skin. With these credentials, it's time to lose that elitist tag and consider this as the leaf of preference for salad basics, where it beautifully combines with an extra virgin olive oil coating to create a strong dual act.

Buckwheat

Buckwheat was one of Japan's first domesticated grains, and the story goes when Buddhist monks took long journeys into the hills, they 'd only bring a clay pot and a buckwheat bag for warmth. Buckwheat is so good that this was all they wanted, and it fed them for weeks. It is one of a sirtuin activator's best-known sources, called rutin. But also, because it has advantages as a cover crop, continuing to improve soil fertility and preventing weed growth, it is a fabulous crop for environmentally sound and sustainable agriculture.

Buckwheat is head and shoulders above most other more growing grains presumably because it's not a grain at all — it's basically a rhubarb-related fruit crop. Holding one of the largest protein contents of any plant, as well as being a sirtfood superpower makes it an unparalleled substitute to more widely used grains. Besides, it's as flexible as any grain and by nature gluten-free, making it a perfect alternative for anyone intolerant to gluten.

Capers

In case you 're not so acquainted with capers, we will discuss those salty, deep green, pellet-like things on top of a pizza that you may only have had opportunity to see. But certainly, they are one of the most undervalued and neglected foods out there. Excitingly, they are the caper bush's flower buds, which emerge extensively in the Mediterranean until collected and stored by hand. Research now shows that capers possess essential antimicrobial, antidiabetic, anti-inflammatory, immunomodulatory, and antimicrobial activities. They have a long tradition of being used as a drug in the Mediterranean and North Africa. It's hardly shocking to find that they are filled with components that trigger sirtuin.

We think it is about time these tiny morsels had their share of fame, much overlooked by the other big hitters of the Mediterranean diet. Flavor-wise, it's a case of huge things coming in little bags, because they're confident they 're kicking it. Even if you don't know how to use them, don't get intimidated. These diminutive nutritional superstars, when provided with the proper ingredients, offer a wonderfully unique and inimitable sour / salty taste to finish off a dish in fashion. They will shortly have you excited and head over heels in love.

Celery

For centuries, Celery was around and admired — with leaves found festooning the ashes of the Egyptian pharaoh Tutankhamun who expired around 1323 BCE. Earlier varieties were very salty, and celery was commonly considered a therapeutic plant particularly for washing and detoxification to prevent disease. It is particularly important considering that liver, kidney, and gut wellbeing are among the other potential effects that research is now showing. In the seventeenth century, it was bred in captivity as a potato and genetic engineering reduced its powerful bitter taste in favor of sweeter types, thereby securing its position as a popular salad vegetable.

It is important to keep in mind that there are two types: blanched/ yellow and Pascal/green. Blanching is a methodology targeted at reducing the typical bitter taste of celery, which has been considered too powerful. This entails filtering the celery before harvesting, contributing to a paler color and a milder flavor. What a tragedy that is, for blanching dumbs down the sirtuin-activating characteristics of celery as well as dumbing down the flavor. Fortunately, the times are changing and people are claiming the actual and unique flavor and backing down to the greener, wide range. Green celery is the type we suggest you use both in green juices and foods, with the heart and leaves being the healthiest pieces.

Chilies

The chili has been an important part of gastronomic culture worldwide for hundreds of years. On one level it's disconcerting that we are so fascinated with it. Its pungent heat, caused by a material called capsaicin, is meant to inflict pain as a plant defensive measure to dissuade predators from feeding on it, and we appreciate that. The food, and our infatuation with it, is now almost magical.

Amazingly, one analysis revealed that consuming chilies together improves cooperation in groups. And from the point of view of health, we realize that the alluring heat is fantastic to activate sirtuins and enhance our metabolic processes. The culinary applications of the chili are limitless, making it very easy to offer a strong sirtfood content to any meal.

While we admire that not everybody is a huge fan of hot or spicy meals, we keep hoping we can help persuade you to simply add small quantities of chilies, following recent studies that suggest that those who eat spicy foods three or more times a week have a fourteen percent lower mortality rate, especially in comparison to those eating them less than once a week.

The spicier the chili, the higher the sirtfood, but be careful and stay with what suits your specific needs. Serrano peppers are a perfect start -they are acceptable for many individuals while packing heat. For more experienced heat seekers, we suggest looking for Thai chilies for full sirtuin-activating advantages. These can be harder to locate in supermarkets but are mostly available in specialized markets in Asia. Search for deep-colored peppers, excluding any with a droopy and fuzzy feel.

Cocoa

It's no great surprise that chocolate was regarded a holy meal for ancient cultures like the Aztecs and Mayans and was typically reserved for the elite and soldiers, served at banquets to achieve allegiance and service. Even so, there was such huge respect for the cocoa bean that it was used as a means of exchange. It was normally served as a frothy beverage back then. What tastier way to get our nutritional allowance of cacao than by chocolate?

Unfortunately, there's no use for the condensed, aged, and chemically-flavored milk chocolate we usually consume. We're talking about chocolate containing 85 percent solids to gain the sirtfood tag. But even then, apart from the amount of cocoa, not all chocolate is made equivalent. To minimize its acidity and give it a darker shade, chocolate is often processed with an alkalizing agent (known as the Dutch process). Regrettably, this reduces the sirtuin-activating flavanols significantly, thus severely undermining its health-promoting efficiency. Luckily, food labeling laws in some countries allow alkalized cocoa to be labelled "alkali produced." Most countries advocate preventing such items. Among greater proportion of cocoa, most preferring those that have not experienced Dutch processing to enjoy the positive effects of cocoa.

Coffee

What's all that about Sirtfood Coffee about? We 're listening to you. We will tell you that there is no mistake. Gone are the days when a pang of shame balanced our pleasure in drinking coffee. Indeed, it is a true treasure trove of wonderful nutrients that activate sirtuin. With more than half of developed countries consuming coffee every day, coffee boasts the honor of being the world's number one source of polyphenols. The biggest irony is that we are admonished by so many fitness "experts" for doing what is in essence the best thing for our wellbeing each day.

This is why coffee lovers have considerably very little diabetes, and reduced costs of some cancers and neurodegenerative diseases. And as the supreme joke, caffeine rather than being a poison positively preserves our livers and makes them safer! Yet counter to the common misconception that coffee dehydrates the body, it is now well known not to be the case, with coffee (and tea) adding well to daily coffee drinkers' liquid intake. And while we understand that coffee is not for everybody and some individuals might be resilient to the negative of caffeine, it's a boon for those who love a cup of tea or coffee.

Extra virgin olive oil

Olive oil is by far the most renowned of Mediterranean dietary staples. The olive tree is one of the oldest recorded domesticated trees, also known as the "immortal tree." Even though people began squeezing olives in stone mortar shells to collect them, the oil had been highly regarded almost 7,000 years earlier. Hippocrates thought it as a cure-all; now, a few millennia later, scientific knowledge categorically asserts its marvelous medical benefits. There is also a plethora of clinical evidence demonstrating that daily olive oil intake is strongly cardioprotective, as well as playing an active role in decreasing the incidence of significant modern-day diseases such as diabetes, other tumors, and osteoporosis. Clearly it is linked to a longer lifespan.

When it comes to olive oil, the trick is to buy additional virgin to receive the benefits of sirtfood in full. Virgin olive oil is only harvested from the fruits by mechanical action that does not contribute to the degradation of the oil, so the consistency and the polyphenol amount can be ensured. "Extra virgin" alludes to the first pressing of the fruit ("virgin" is the second pressing). It has the best taste, effectiveness, and strongest credentials of sirtfood, and is therefore the one that we highly suggest in your diet.

Garlic

Garlic has been regarded one of Nature's miracle foods for hundreds of years, with soothing and rejuvenating properties. Egyptians fed pyramid crews with garlic to increase their immune response, discourage various diseases, and enhance their potential to suppress fatigue. Garlic is a potent natural antibiotic and antifungal that is sometimes used to help cure ulcers in the stomach. By accelerating the withdrawal of metabolic waste products, it can encourage the lymphatic system to "detox." So, despite being tested for weight reduction, it also delivers a powerful heart safety punch, decreasing cholesterol by around ten percent and reducing blood pressure by five to seven percent, as well as decreasing the stickiness of the blood. So, if you are concerned about the taste of garlic being off-putting, be aware. When women were asked to determine a range of men's body odors, it was found that all men who ate four or more garlic cloves a day had a much more appealing and friendly smell. Experts suggest this is because it is regarded as a strong signal of wellbeing.

The sirtfood nutrients in garlic are enhanced by another main nutrient called allicin that gives it its distinctive fragrance. But only after physical "harm" to the bulb does allicin develops in garlic. So, when subject to temperature (cooking) or poor pH (stomach acid), its composition is halted. So, when preparing garlic, chop, thin, or crush it and then allow the mixture to rest for about ten minutes prior to actually cooking or eating.

Green tea (Especially matcha)

Many are experienced with green tea, the toast of the Orient and ever more famous in the West. Public consciousness knows its medical benefits; green tea consumption is linked to less cancer, heart disease, kidney disease and osteoporosis. The explanation is that green tea is so healthy for us largely due to its valuable content of a group of effective plant compounds called catechins. The center of attention is a special form of sirtuin-activating catechin identified as epigallocatechin gallate (EGCG).

What's the debate about matcha, though? We like to think of matcha as steroids in ordinary green tea. In comparison to traditional green tea, which is processed as an infusion, it is a unique powdered green tea formulated by dissolving completely in water. The upshot of consuming matcha is that it comprises significantly higher levels of the sirtuin-activating component EGCG than other green teas. Matcha is defined as the "absolute mentally and physically cure with the potential to make one's life completely full" if you are seeking for more encouragement.

Kale

We are cynics at heart and are still suspicious of what is causing the new craze for health food ads. Is it science, or are other interests involved? In recent times, few foods have boomed as significantly as kale on the wellbeing scene. Explained as the "lean, green brassica queen" (making reference to its cruciferous vegetable family), this has become the chic vegetable for which all health-lovers and food bloggers are gearing up. Every October there is also a National Day of the Kale. But you don't have to wait until then to express your kale joy: there are already T-shirts, featuring trendy slogans like "Driven by Kale" and "Road to Kale." This is enough for us to hear the warning bells.

We've done extensive research, filled with concerns, and we have to acknowledge that our result is that kale really deserves her pleasures (even though we still don't suggest the T-shirts!). The explanation why we're pro-kale is that it contains bumper numbers of quercetin and kaempferol sirtuin-activating compounds, rendering it a have to-include in the Sirtfood Diet as the source of our green sirtfood drink. What's so exciting about kale is that the curly vegetable is accessible anywhere, produced locally and very inexpensive, unlike most of the typical expensive, hard-to-source, and hugely overpriced so-called superfoods!

Medjool dates

It may come as a shock to include Medjool dates in a collection of foods that encourage weight loss and good health—especially when we inform you that Medjool dates comprise a whopping 66 percent sugar. Sugar doesn't have any sirtuin-activating qualities at all; rather, it has established links to obesity, heart disease, and diabetes — just the reverse of what we're looking to accomplish. But processed foods' sugar is very distinct from sugar taken in a naturally-supplied vehicle aligned with sirtuin-activating polyphenols: the date of the Medjool.

Medjool dates, consumed in moderation, do not really have any significant blood-sugar-raising impacts, in absolute comparison with regular sugar. Consuming them is related to fewer diabetes and cardiac disorders. They have been a staple food worldwide for decades, and there has been an increase in medical interest in dates in recent times, which sees them rising as a possible remedy for a variety of diseases. It is where the Sirtfood Diet 's beauty and strength lie. It refutes existing dogma and helps you to engage in a nice treat in moderation.

Parsley

Parsley is a cooking conundrum. It often appears in dishes, and it's the only green guy too often. At best we serve a few chopped sprigs as an afterthought on a plate, at worst a single sprig for festive reasons only. It is sadly languishing on the plate even after we have stopped eating. This foodie styling trend stems from its conventional use in ancient Rome as a side dish for eating after meals to refresh the palate, rather than being part of the meal itself. And what an embarrassment, because parsley is an amazing food that packs a vibrant, delicious flavor full of character.

Besides that, what makes parsley really special is that it is an essential source of sirtuin-activating nutrient apigenin, a tremendous blessing because it is found only in large quantities in other foods. Apigenin attaches wondrously to the benzodiazepine receptors in our brains, enabling us to calm down and rest. It's time we enjoyed parsley not as an omnipresent dietary confetto but as a result of our own choice to achieve the wonderful medical advantages it can offer.

Red endive

Endive is a fairly new kid on the block in so far as vegetables go. History has it that a Belgian farmer found endive in 1830 by mistake. The farmer processed chicory roots in his storeroom and then used them as a sort of coffee substitute, only to overlook them. Upon his arrival he noticed that white leaves had started growing, which he considered to be soft, crunchy, and very tasty upon eating. Endive is grown throughout the world, such as the US and earns its sirtfood tag thanks to its remarkable sirtuin enhancer, luteolin material. And besides the proven sirtuin-activating effects, luteolin intake has become an effective therapy option to improve socialization in autistic children.

It has a pleasing appearance and a sweet taste for those new to endive, followed by a gentle and friendly bitterness. If you want boost endive in a meal, you can't lose by having her foliage to a salad where its welcome, tart flavor adds a great zesty bite with an extra virgin olive oil coating. Red is great, much like onion, but the yellow kind can also be called a sirtfood. Whereas the red range may sometimes be more challenging to find, we can absolutely guarantee that yellow is an entirely acceptable substitute.

Red onions

Since the time of our prehistoric ancestors, onions have been a super food, one of the first vegetables to be grown around 5,000 years ago. For such a lengthy tradition of use and such strong health-giving qualities, many societies before us have honored onions. They were held in esteem particularly by the Egyptians as subjects of devotion, considering their circle-within-a-circle form is indicative of eternal afterlife. And the Greeks assumed that onions made athletes stronger. Athletes would eat their way through large quantities of onions before the games, even drinking the juice! It's an amazing testament to how important traditional dietary knowledge can be when we remember that onions deserve their place in the top 20 sirtfood foods. They're chock-full of the sirtuin-activating compounds quercetin — the very component that the sports science industry has recently started aggressively studying and promoting to boost athletic performance.

Why the red ones? Obviously because they have a higher concentration of quercetin, but the regular yellow ones do not fall far behind and also offer a great selection.

Red wine

The top twenty sirtfoods are complete without the addition of the original sirtfood, red wine. The French phenomenon gained notoriety in the early 1990s. Despite the French doing things wrong when it came to wellbeing (cigarettes, lack of physical activity, and expensive eating habits), they had lower death rates from cardiovascular disease than countries like the United States. The justification for as recommended by doctors was the extensive amount of red wine they drink. Danish research teams in 1995 illustrated that a low-to-moderate usage of red wine decreased mortality rate, whereas roughly the same level of beverage alcohol had no impact. And a comparable consumption of hard liquors continues to increase mortality rate. Obviously, in 2003, the fertile quality of red wine with a bevy of sirtuin-activating components was discovered, and the rest, as they claim, was history.

One 5-ounce drink a day for females and up to two 5-ounce drinks a day for males falls within US standards. Wines from the many regions (especially pinot noir, cabernet sauvignon, and merlot) have the maximum polyphenol content among the most commonly accessible wines to guarantee the most sirtuin-activating bang for your buck.

Soy

Soy products have a long tradition as an important part of a healthy diet of many nations in Asia-Pacific such as China, Japan, and Korea. Research teams first became switched on to soy after discovering that high soy-consuming countries had considerably lower incidences of many cancers, particularly breast and prostate cancers. It is believed to be due to a special class of polyphenols found in soybeans known as isoflavones that can positively affect how estrogens function in the body - that include the daidzein and formononetin sirtuin-activators. Soy oil intake has also been related to a decrease in the occurrence or intensity of a number of diseases such as heart disease, the effects of menopause and bone loss.

Highly refined, nutritionally-stripped soybean formulations are now a common component in various packaged foods. The advantages are gained either from actual soy products such as tofu, an outstanding provider of vegan protein, or in fortified form such as tempeh, natto, or our favorite, miso, a typical Japanese paste fortified with a naturally present fungus that results in an extreme umami taste.

Strawberries

In recent times, fruit has been particularly vilified, having a poor reputation amid the rising fervor for sugar. Luckily, such a malignant image couldn't be more undeserved for berry-lovers. Although all berries are giants of protein, strawberries are winning their 20 largest sirtfood status owing to their excess of the fisetin sirtuin activator. And now research advocates daily eating of strawberries to encourage health and longevity, staving off Alzheimer's, obesity, diabetes, cardiovascular disease, and osteoporosis. As for their nutritional value, a mere tablespoon per 3 1/2 ounces is very small.

Amusingly, intrinsically low in sugar, strawberries have a special way for the body to respond to carbohydrates. Studies have discovered that adding strawberries to carbohydrates decreases the need for insulin, effectively transforming a meal into a constant sugar releaser. Recent work also shows that consuming strawberries for diabetes treatment has results close to opioid therapy.

Turmeric

Turmeric, a derivative of ginger, is the latest kid on the health food block. While we are just switching to it now here in the West, it has been valued for hundreds of years in Asia, for both its nutritional and therapeutic applications. Amazingly, India generates almost the entire world's turmeric supply, eating 80 % of the total itself. In Asia, turmeric is used to treat skin diseases like acne, psoriasis, skin irritation and rash. Prior to Indian weddings, there is a celebration where turmeric paste is used as a skin skincare routine for the bride and groom and also to ward off misery.

One factor that prevents turmeric's potency is that the main sirtuin-activating compound, curcumin, is poorly absorbed into the body when we consume it. Research, however, reveals that we can overcome this by preparing it in a liquid, introducing fat and black pepper to boost its uptake significantly. This fits well within Indian cuisine, where ghee and black pepper are traditionally mixed in sauces and other hot dishes, once again proving that research matches up with the age-old experience of conventional methods.

Walnuts

Going all the way back to 7000 BCE, walnuts are the world's oldest manmade tree product, emerging in ancient Persia where they were the property of the nobility. Fast forward to the present day, and walnuts are a big success in the US. California is leading the way, with its Central Valley famous as the prime walnut-growing area. California walnuts also provide the United States with ninety percent of market production and a whopping three-quarters of nationwide production.

Walnut are the number one nut for wellbeing. What makes walnuts stand out is how they add to mainstream wisdom: they are high in nutrients and are well-established for weight reduction and fighting off the threat of biochemical diseases such as heart disease and diabetes. This is the strength of activating the sirtuin.

Recent literature revealing walnuts to be an effective anti-aging nutrient is less well known but equally fascinating. Evidence refers to their advantages as a brain food with the ability to slow down brain aging and lower the risk of debilitating brain diseases, as well as reducing mounting deterioration from physical activity over time.

DIET BOOSTING FOODS

Avocado

Protein amount	Quantity of product
2 g	Each half avocado

This fruit contains all 9 essential amino acids, plus cardiac omega-3 fatty acids.

Milk

Protein amount	Quantity of product
9-10 g	One cup

Milk makes for a healthy body, really. As well as packaging plenty of protein, milk is also a great source of nutrients that build bones.

Cheese

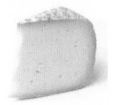

Protein amount	Quantity of product
7 g	1 ounce

Yeah, cheese can be part of a balanced diet — until you overindulge. Adhere to a serving size and combine it with an apple for an ultra-healthy appetizer.

Tempeh

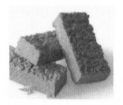

Protein amount	Quantity of product
15 g	Half cup

The Kit Kat bar-like texture makes the seitan a stand-in for smart meat. Salt it over salads, or with chopped tempeh.

Asparagus

Protein amount	Quantity of product
4 g	One cup

This tasty veggie is a powerhouse of nutrients. Enjoy it steamed or grilled, or scatter seeds in salads.

Black beans

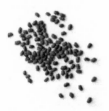

Protein amount	Quantity of product
7-9 g	Half cup

Enlist black beans with rice or quinoa for a full protein meal.

Lentils

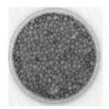

Protein amount	Quantity of product
9 g	½ cup

Nutritionist, Marjorie Nolan Cohn, the New York City owner of MNC Nutrition, reaches for foods high in resistant starch, a special fiber type. "The small intestine does not digest resistant starch, meaning it reaches the whole of the large intestine where it ferments," she says. "This method involves beneficial fatty acids that might obstruct a person's ability to burn carbohydrates and, instead, it uses recently eaten stored body fat as fuel."

Greek yogurt

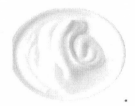

Protein amount	Quantity of product
18 g	6 oz

This rich and creamy treat contains almost twice as much protein as other sources of milk; it is perfect with fruit.

Tree nuts

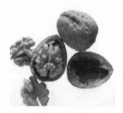

Protein amount	Quantity of product
4-6 g	2 tablespoons

A pound of walnuts or almonds is great as a sweet treat, mixed with yogurt or in a salad.

Edamame

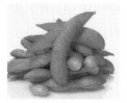

Protein amount	Quantity of product
8.5 g	Half cup

In individually packaged packs is almost every trace of mineral needed by your body, including iron, magnesium, and zinc.

Whey protein

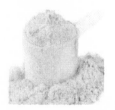

Protein amount	Quantity of product
24 g	1 oz

For a fast protein hit, add a scoop to smoothies or water. Try protein powder in soy.

Spinach

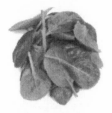

Protein amount	Quantity of product
5 g	1 cup (cooked)

Spinach boasts the highest protein content of all the leafy greens. Try sautéing it with a little garlic.

Tofu

Protein amount	Quantity of product
12 g	3 oz

This low-calorie, flexible protein is made from soybeans and will take on any flavor, from Asian to barbecue.

Fish and shellfish

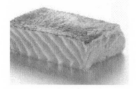

Protein amount	Quantity of product
28 g	4 oz

Seafood is a great catch, whether salmon, halibut or tuna. Target 3 to 5 servings per week.

Pseudo grains

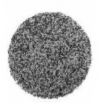

Protein amount	Quantity of product
5-9 g	1 cup(cooked)

These hearty, grainy seeds (quinoa, amaranth, and buckwheat) contain more protein than conventional wheat.

Chickpeas

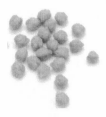

Protein amount	Quantity of product
15 g	1 cup

Eat them as a snack, add them to a salad or throw them in the food processor per a nice hummus recipe.

Eggs

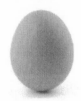

Protein amount	Quantity of product
12 g	2 eggs
14 g	4 white eggs

Eggs and egg whites are smart food for muscles however you prepare them. (Take a look at our healthy morning breakfasts ideas.)

Poultry and pork

Protein amount	Quantity of product
28 g	4 oz

Family faves like skinless chicken and pork make every meal easy to score enough protein.

Hemp seeds

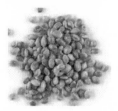

Protein amount	Quantity of product
11 g	3 tablespoons

Sprinkle the hemp seeds on rice, smoothies, or salads for an extra crunch.

Cottage cheese

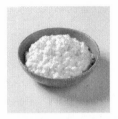

Protein amount	Quantity of product
25 g	1 cup

For a sweet and satisfying breakfast combine cottage cheese with berries or pineapple. A word of warning: cottage cheese can be high in sodium, so carefully read the label.

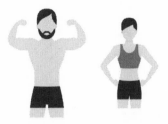

Chapter 4:
How to Build Muscle

O
ne surprising result from our own study that really puzzled us was that the respondents' muscle mass did not drop; instead, it rose by just over one pound on average. Although it was normal at seven pounds, we saw something interesting happening too. The losses in body measurements were disheartening for just about two-thirds of our attendees, while still very remarkable, with a weight reduction of just over five lbs. But when experiments were conducted on body shape, we were astonished. The attendees' muscle mass was not only maintained, but it was enhanced. The total muscle growth for this category was almost two

pounds, adding seven pounds to what is called the "muscular gain based losing weight."

This was totally shocking and in marked contrast to what usually occurs on diets for weight-loss, where individuals lose some fat but also lose muscle strength. For any diet that reduces kcal, it's the traditional trade-off: you say good-bye muscles and also fat. It is not at all shocking when you know that cells change from their growth phase to defense mode as we starve the body of nutrition, causing protein from muscles to be used as food.

SIRTUINS AND MUSCLE MASS

Within the body, a group of genes function as defenders of our muscles when undergoing stress to avoid collapse: these are sirtuins. SIRT1 is a strong Muscle Degradation Antagonist. As long as SIRT1 is triggered, muscle deterioration is stopped even when we're fasting, so we start to burn fat for energy.

But SIRT1 's advantages aren't limited to maintaining lean muscle. In fact, sirtuins improve and increase skeletal muscle strength and mass. We ought to delve into the fascinating world of stem cells to illustrate how the process works. Our muscles exhibit a particular form of stem cell called a satellite cell that regulates its development and reconstruction. Much of the time, satellite cells just sit in silence, but they are powered up when muscle get damaged or stressed. Through weightlifting and similar activities, our muscles grow stronger. SIRT1 is important for triggering satellite cells, so muscles are considerably weaker without their operation since they no longer have the ability to fully grow or repair. Even then, we are giving more power to our satellite cells by raising SIRT1 activation to promote muscle growth and repair.

SIRTFOODS VERSUS FASTING

A major question arises: if activation of sirtuin enhances muscle strength, why do we lose more muscle when we fast? Fasting also stimulates our sirtuin genes, one of fasting's big advantages.

Not all structural muscles are equal. There are two key forms: type-1 and type-2 surprisingly. The type-1 muscle is used for movements for prolonged periods, while type-2 muscles are used for brief periods with more strenuous exercise. Here it gets fascinating: fasting tends to increase SIRT1 action in muscle fibers type-1, not type-2. So, the size of type-1 muscle fiber is preserved and even increases exponentially if we are fasting. Unfortunately, in absolute comparison to what occurs throughout fasting in type-1 fibers, SIRT1 decreases quickly in type-2 fibers. This indicates the fat burning comes to a halt, and muscles break down to provide heat.

For muscles tissues, fasting will be a double-edged sword, with type-2 fibers getting a kick. Type-2 fibers make up the bulk of our muscles. But though our type-1 fiber mass is increasing with fasting we still see a substantial and expected loss of muscles. If we were to avoid muscle collapse, it would not only make us look healthy but also hopefully encourage more weight loss. And the way to do this is to fight the drop in SIRT1 in muscle fiber type-2 caused by fasting.

Scientists brought this to the test in an interesting mice trial and found that throughout fasting, the triggers for glycogen depletion were turned off by inducing SIRT1 activity in type-2 fibers such that no muscle damage occurred.

The investigators then took a step forward and checked the impact on mice musculature of elevated SIRT1 activation when the mice were fed rather than felt hungry and found that it caused very massive muscle development. In a week, muscle cells with elevated levels of SIRT1 activation displayed an impressive weight gain of twenty percent.

These research results are comparable to the end result of our Sirtfood Diet trial, although in impact, our study has been relatively mild. By enhancing SIRT1 activity and consuming a diet rich in sirtfoods, most respondents had no muscle damage — and for others, just a mild strong muscle mass was shown.

KEEPING MUSCLES YOUNG

This is not just about the tone and appearance of the body. SIRT1 's extensive impact on the body affects the way it operates too. When a muscle ages it loses its capacity to trigger SIRT1. This renders it less sensitive to workout effects and more vulnerable to reactive oxygen species and inflammatory destruction, resulting in what is known as oxidative stress. Progressively, muscles become weaker, making the individual more easily tired. But if we can boost SIRT1 activation, we can prevent the downward trend associated with aging.

Nevertheless, through triggering SIRT1 to avoid the loss of muscle mass and activity we usually associate with aging, we see several different medical benefits, like arresting bone loss and avoiding chronic systemic inflammation (known as inflammation), along with increased agility and improved general quality of life. So, interestingly, our new study shows that the higher the polyphenol level (and hence sirtuin-activating nutrients) in older individuals' diets, the more they ward off deteriorating physical activity with aging.

Don't be misled into believing that such incentives extend only to the aged; far from that. Around the age of twenty-five, the symptoms of aging begin, and muscles gradually decline by ten percent by the age of forty (although average weight continues to increase) with a loss of forty percent by age 70. Yet there is considerable evidence that the activation of our sirtuin genes will inhibit and undo all of this.

In loss of muscle development, sirtuin activity plays a crucial role. Pile it on and it's no surprise that sirtuins are present in muscle building according to a recent analysis in the prestigious medical journal, Nature. The study cites rising sirtuin stimulation as one of the faster avenues for battling loss of muscle mass, thereby increasing quality of life while lessening illness and mortality.

Considering the strong impact sirtuin genetics can have on muscles, our prototype trial's surprise findings no longer appeared so surprising. We began to realize that spurring weight loss while trying to feed our muscle groups was feasible, all through a balanced diet in sirtfood.

But this is only the beginning. We'll discuss sirtfoods' advantages much more as they apply to all facets of health and wellbeing.

SUMMARY

- Even after weight loss we find that individuals either retain or add muscles during the Sirtfood Diet. This is because sirtuins are the chief muscle controllers.
- By triggering the sirtuins, muscle collapse can be prevented and muscle restoration promoted.

- SIRT1 activation can also assist in avoiding the significant deterioration of muscles that we see with aging.
- Triggering your sirtuin genetics will not only make you appear leaner but will also help you remain healthy and productive as you mature.

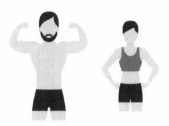

Chapter 5:

How to Build a Diet That Works

TIPS TO BUILD THE SIRTFOOD DIET THAT BETTER SUITS YOU

We have done something very unique with the Sirtfood Diet. We took the most powerful sirtfoods in the biosphere and have woven them into a brand-new healthy diet, the likes of which have not been seen before. We picked the "best and brightest" from the best-known healthful diets and have built tried and true recipes of our own.

The great thing is that you don't immediately have to follow an Okinawan's typical diet or eat like an Italian mamma. On the Sirtfood Diet this is not only utterly infeasible, but also needless. One thing you may notice from sirtfoods list is their similarity. While you may not be consuming some of the items on the list at the moment, you are probably eating others. So why don't you just lose weight already?

The issue is addressed when we analyze the cutting-edge nutrition science now displays as required to build a workable diet. It is about eating proper amount of sirtfoods. It's about adding ample protein portions to sirtfood bowls, and then enjoying your food at the right time of day. And it's about the freedom to eat the genuinely savory foods you love in the quantities you desire.

HITTING YOUR QUOTA

Most people don't eat nearly enough sirtfoods to get a strong fat-burning and fitness-boosting benefit. When we looked at the consumption in the US of the five main sirtuin-activating components (quercetin, luteolin, myricetin, kaempferol, and apigenin), human dietary intake was found to be a miserable thirteen milligrams a day. Conversely, the Japanese daily consumption is 5 times greater. Contrast that with our Sirtfood Diet experiment, where every day the subjects ate hundreds of milligrams of sirtuin-activating foods.

We are speaking about a true diet transformation in which we raise our daily consumption of sirtuin-activating components by as much as 50 times. Although that might seem overwhelming or unrealistic, it isn't at all. By taking all your highest level sirtfoods and putting them together in a manner fully consistent with your typical stressful schedule, you can efficiently and economically reach the level needed to gain all known advantages.

THE POWER OF SYNERGY

We think it is important to eat a vast array of these wonder nutrients as organic whole foods, where they coexist along with dozens of other natural biologically active substances that work synergistically to increase our wellbeing. We think working with the natural world is best, instead of against. Single nutrient supplementation does not display permanent effects time after time, but the same component is represented in an entire diet.

Take, for example, the basic component, resveratrol, that activates sirtuin. It is partially consumed in supplementary form, but its bioavailability (how much more the individual can use) is at least 6 times higher in the normal food content of red wine. Red wine produces not only one but a complete variety of sirtuin-activating polyphenols that work with each other to produce positive effects like myricetin, piceatannol, quercetin and epicatechin. Perhaps we should direct our focus from turmeric to curcumin. Curcumin is well-established as the main sirtuin-activating ingredient in turmeric, but studies reveals that whole turmeric has stronger PPAR-ÿ action to combat fat burning and is much more capable of suppressing cancer and decreasing blood glucose levels than isolated curcumin. It's not hard to understand that isolating a single nutrient is still nowhere near as successful as eating it.

Combining multiple sirtfoods is what really makes a nutritional plan special. For example, by introducing it in quercetin-rich sirtfoods, we enhance the impact of resveratrol-containing foods a lot more. They complement one another. They are all fat blockers, but how either actually achieves this is complicated. Resveratrol is very effective in promoting the deterioration of mature fat cells, while quercetin is active in preventing new fat tissue from developing. In addition, they ingest food on both ends, leading to a high weight loss impact more than consuming just large amounts of a single ingredient.

This is a method we are beginning to see again and again. Foods high in sirtuin boost quercetin uptake from one's diet and increase its function. Quercetin in effect has been shown to be synergistic with epigallocatechin gallate (EGCG) activity. And EGCG 's work with curcumin has been seen to be complementary. And so it begins. Not only are individual whole products more effective than single ingredients, but we reach into another tapestry of beneficial effects that the natural world has woven — so deep and so pure, it's difficult to beat it.

JUICING AND FOOD: GET THE BEST OF BOTH WORLDS

The Sirtfood Diet comprises both juices and whole food products. We are speaking about juices made directly from a juicer. Blenders and milkshake makers (including the NutriBullet) do not work. That may sound counterintuitive, but fiber is lost during juicing, just what we need from leafy green vegetables.

Fiber includes what is termed non-extractable polyphenols (or NEPPs). Polyphenols, called sirtuin additives, are bound to the fibrous portion of food and only emitted by our helpful intestinal bacteria when decomposed. We don't even get NEPPs by suppressing fiber and end up losing out. Crucially, though, the NEPP composition varies significantly based on the size of the plant. The NEPP material of a diet rich in fruits, cereals, and grains is meaningful and should be ingested whole (NEPPs provide over fifty percent of polyphenols in strawberries!). However, as for leafy green vegetables, the essential compounds in sirtfood juice, they are much less even than a bigger fiber content.

So, we get full bang for our buck when we juice leafy green vegetables and eliminating the low-nutrient material. We can even use increasing quantities and obtain an amazingly concentrated dose of sirtuin-activating polyphenols.

There is yet another benefit of cutting the fiber, too. Green leafy vegetables contain a form of fiber called non-soluble fiber which has a gastrointestinal scrubbing action. However, when we consume so much of it, it will frustrate and hurt our digestive lining like when we over-scrub stuff. For so many people, green leafy vegetables-packed smoothies can overwhelm fiber, possibly aggravating or even inducing IBS (irritable bowel syndrome) and hampering our nutrient uptake.

When it comes to digesting their goodness, having a few of your sirtfoods in juice form can have significant benefits. For instance, matcha green tea is one of the additives we include in green juice. When we drink the EGCG sirtuin activator present in high amounts of green tea in the form of drinks lacking milk, its ingestion is higher than sixty-five percent. We also found that it is important to remember that transitioning from smoothies to green juices carries a significant rise in quantities of other vital nutrients, including such magnesium and folic acid.

The core issue is that to get those sirtuin genetic factors working for massive weight loss and wellbeing, we have to establish an eating plan that incorporates both juices and whole meals.

THE POWER OF PROTEIN

There are plants that bring the sirt in sirtfood; to get optimum value, sirtfood foods must have a high protein content. A major component of the dietary specific protein, leucine, has extra advantages in enhancing SIRT1 to activate fat loss and boost blood sugar regulation.

But leucine has another role, where it genuinely glows through its balanced interaction with sirtfoods. Leucine effectively induces anabolism (building things) in our cells, especially in muscles, which requires a great deal of energy causing our energy producers (called mitochondria) to work extra hours. This induces the need for a sirtfoods operation within our cells. As you may remember, one of the impacts of sirtfoods is to increase the growth of more mitochondria, to increase their efficiency, and to make them use fat as fuel. Our bodies therefore need them to fulfill this extra demand for energy. The truth of the matter is that we see a synergistic impact when mixing sirtfoods with dietary protein that will enhance sirtuin activation and eventually allow you to lose fat to support muscle development and safety. For this reason the meals in this guide are designed to contain a reasonable protein portion.

Oily fish are an incredibly strong protein alternative to supplement sirtfoods' action since they are high in omega-3 fatty acids alongside their nutritional value. There is no way you haven't read a lot about the health effects of oily fish and especially omega-3 fish oils. Now new evidence shows that the advantages of omega-3 fats may come from improving the functioning of our sirtuin genomes.

In recent times, questions have been raised about the harmful impact of protein-rich diets on wellbeing; without any sirtfoods to help counter the protein, we can recognize why. Leucine may be a sword with two-edges. We need sirtfoods, as we have shown, to support our cells fulfill the metabolic requirements that leucine imposes upon them. Without them, though, our mitochondria may become unstable, so elevated rates of leucine will potentially encourage obesity and insulin tolerance, rather than boost safety. Sirtfoods not only keep the symptoms of leucine in control but also work effectively in our favor. Assume leucine as pressing your foot on the losing weight and wellbeing accelerator, with sirtfoods the device guaranteeing that the cells fulfill the increased competition. The engine blow ups without any sirtfoods.

Returning to worries about the safety consequences of protein-rich diets, the missing part of the equation is sirtfoods. Usually, most nations' diets are protein-rich but lack sirtfoods to help counter it. That makes it imperative for sirtfoods becoming an essential component of how these nations consume nutrition.

EAT EARLY

Our ideology is that relatively earlier is superior when it comes to having a meal, preferably completing eating each day by 7 p.m. That is on two grounds. First, to enjoy the sirtfoods' natural satiating power. Eating food that will leave you feeling full, happy, and energetic as you go about your day is even more effective than enduring the whole day feeling hungry enough to eat and staying full while sleeping throughout the night.

Yet there's a second good explanation to maintain dietary behaviors in line with your own body clock. We all have an internal body clock, called our circadian clock, which controls all of our normal functioning. It affects, inter alia, how the body processes the food we eat. Our clocks work in synchronization, above all trying to follow the signs of the sun's light-dark cycle. We 're programmed as a diurnal organism to be effective in the daylight rather than at nighttime. Our body clock therefore permits us to operate most effectively during the day. Whenever it's light, we're intended to be active, and far less so when it's dark, when we're preparing for proper sleep.

The question is that all of us have "work clocks" and "social clocks," which are not aligned with the sun's waning. After dusk is the last option any of us get to sleep. To some extent, we can equip our circadian rhythm to synchronize with rotating shifts, like "evening chronotypes" that can be effective if we eat properly and sleep later in the day. People who lives out of the light-dark exterior cycle know that it comes with a price. Research shows that people in the evening chronotype have an increased susceptibility to gain body fat, muscle atrophy and metabolic disorders, as well as often having sleep deprivation. That's precisely what we see in night shift workers, who probably have a higher prevalence of obesity and metabolic disorders, at least partly due to the impact of their delayed dietary behaviors.

The fact of the matter is that where necessary, you 're best off eating early in the day, preferably by 7 p.m. But what if it is not possible? The great news is that sirtuins play a key part in synchronizing the circadian rhythm. Studies have shown that the polyphenols in sirtfoods are able to modulate our body rhythms and change the circadian rhythm favorably. This implies the addition of sirtfoods into your meals will mitigate the adverse consequences if you cannot stop consuming food late. Evidently, one of the recurring reviews we hear from Sirtfood Diet supporters is how often their sleep patterns have continued to improve, suggesting a significant effect on body clock harmonization.

GO BIG ON TASTE

A basic problem with current our eating habits is that the eating experience is often uncomfortable. They flushes away every little drop of food enjoyment, leaving us feeling bitter. But it's important that in maintaining a healthier weight you retain the pleasure of food. That's why we were happy when we noticed that sirtfoods and the food products that improve their action like protein and omega-3 sources of food are prepared to satisfy our flavor buds. It's an overall win-win: the Sirtfood Diet boosts our wellbeing while imparting wonderful tastes.

Let's go back to see how all this works. Our sense of taste evaluates how tasty we find our food, and how comfortable we are to consume it. This is accomplished by the 7 main receptors of taste. Human beings have developed over hundreds of generations to pursue the flavors that enhance these receptors to reach optimal nutrition out of our diet. The more these flavor receptors are activated by a food, the more pleasure we get from a meal. So, we have the perfect list to satisfy the sense of taste in our Sirtfood Diet. It delivers a full affect to our picky taste receptors. To reveal the foods you'll eat on the diet menu, we include the 7 major sensations of taste: sweet (strawberries, dates); sour (strawberries); bitter (cocoa, kale, extra virgin olive oil, endive green tea); stingy (chilies, garlic, extra virgin olive oil); salty (celery, fish); astringent (green tea, red wine); and umami (soy, fish, meat).

We have found that the higher a food's sirtuin-activating entities, the stronger it enhances our flavor centers, and the more satisfaction we get from the food we consume. Crucially, it also ensures that our hunger is met sooner and our urge to consume more is appropriate. That is a primary explanation why those eating a sirtfood-rich diet are fuller faster.

Organic cocoa, for instance, has an enticing sour aftertaste, but it is superior to the sirtuin-activating flavanols in industrial food products. We've decided to leave behind the density-produced, uninteresting, and charmless cocoa used to make overly sweet chocolate pastries. The beneficial effects have disappeared by this point.

The same is true of olive oil. In its moderately refined form — extra virgin — it has a strong and unique taste that can be sensed at the back of the tongue. Yet refined and processed olive oil starts to lose its punch; it is tasteless and does not carry a kick . Likewise, hot chilies hold much more sirtuin-activating credibility than the relatively mild kinds, and wild strawberries are much tastier than the domesticated ones due to their stronger sirtuin-activating nutritional value.

Specific sirtfoods can stimulate various receptors of flavor: green tea is both unpleasant and astringent, and strawberries combine sweet and savory flavors. At first, some palates won't get used to some of these flavors as much of our industrial diets is devoid both of nutrients and genuine taste — but you'd be surprised at how fast you gain affection for them. Besides, humans are wired to look for a healthy diet in sirtfoods, along with healthy protein and omega-3 fatty acids, to gratify our basic instincts and, in turn, our wellbeing. The process of evolution has been going on for millennia without us understanding the cause, yet it has guaranteed that we get the greatest return from eating such foods.

EMBRACE EATING

Let's try an experiment. We want you to do one very easy thing for us: don't dream about a polar bear. What do you think? Of course, a polar bear. Why? For what? Even though we told you not to. Don't tell us you're still going to think about them!

It was the innovating survey conducted in 1987 by psychology professor, Daniel Wegner, that revealed that the compelled repression of thought leads to a contradictory and ineffective intensification of what we are attempting to suppress. So rather than obstructing our thought processes, the activity generates a focus on the inhibited thought.

The very same thing occurs when we are antagonists to weight-loss diet products. Research shows that in fact we have assumptions about them, increasing our interest. There are dozens of fads like chewing before swallowing, plus the escalating anxiety over "forbidden" foods.

Scientists have clarified what's going on here. We need to be fully autonomous. When we feel restricted, like going on a limited diet, it causes a bad feeling that makes us feel uncomfortable. We get wrapped up in our misery and fight to get out. We take up arms by doing what we've been told we shouldn't be doing and a lot more than we would have had at first. It happens with everyone, even the most self-controlled. It's not a case of when, but if. Think about bingers. Researchers now agree that while we can sustain certain foods and understand the benefits, we still struggle to achieve long-term progress.

Does this mean that there is no sense in trying to improve our food patterns? Are we just doomed to fail? Yes, we need to make our own optimistic, ideal decisions to be successful. We now know that it is not through nutritional isolation but through dietary inclusion. Rather than concentrating your energy on the negative aspects of what you shouldn't eat, conversely look at the positive aspects of what you should eat. The Sirtfood Diet's elegance is in this. It's about what you include in your meal and not what you throw out. It is about the reliability and not the amount consumed. It's about desiring to do something because you feel fulfilled eating great-tasting food with the knowledge that every chomp provides a treasure trove of advantages.

Many diets are a means to an end. They're about trying to make sense of the "thin dream." However, at the end of the day, it never happens and the diet fails, so it's never maintained. Now there is a special Sirtfood Diet. Phase 1 reduces calories, deliberately short and quick to ensure positive effects before an adverse reaction happens. The emphasis is exclusively on sirtfoods. So, the desire to eat sirtfoods isn't just motivated by the end goal of weight loss. Now it's about appreciating and celebrating natural food for a safe and healthy lifestyle.

What's more, once you gain sirtfoods' useful benefits, from satisfying your desire to enhancing your quality of life, you'll find your habits and tastes vary. On the Sirtfood Diet, items that would have traditionally set off a chain of adverse responses (especially if taboo) find their attraction wanes. They now become a small component of a balanced diet and accomplished without a random bear sighting.

SUMMARY

- The Sirtfood Diet draws on the earth's most effective sirtfoods and puts them together in an easy and realistic way.

- To obtain optimum performance, lose weight and attain wellbeing, sirtfoods should be consumed in the correct amount, mixture, and formulation to achieve the stimulatory activity of their sirtuin-activating chemicals.

- We further improve this by including quality foods such as leucine-rich protein sources and oily fish, to start making the Sirtfood Diet's impacts even more potent.

- Nutrition early in the day is also vital and generally keeps us in sync with our built-in circadian rhythm.

- Unlike traditional diets, sirtfoods satisfy our sweet tooth, meaning that we get more pleasure from our meals and feel satisfied quicker.

- The Sirtfood Diet is a participation diet – not a restriction diet and the only diet that can result in long-term weight-loss achievement.

PHASE 1: 7 POUNDS IN SEVEN DAYS

This is a step in the direction of high energy-success toward accomplishing a thinner and slimmer body. Following our easy step-by-step directions and enjoy the tasty meals you'll make. We have a meat-free option in comparison to our regular seven-day schedule ideal for vegetarians and vegans alike. Go with whatever you prefer.

WHAT TO EXPECT

You'll receive the amazing rewards of our scientifically-validated strategy of losing seven pounds in seven days during the initiation phase. It involves adding strength, so don't just get caught up on measurements. Nor should you become accustomed to weighing yourself every day. In reality, over the last few days of Phase 1, we always see the scales starting to creep up in number due to muscle tone, while our waists continue to dwindle in size. Therefore, focus on the scales, but don't be governed by them. Find out how you feel when your clothes fit, or when you need to push another notch in your belt. These are excellent examples of the deeper adjustments expected in body makeup.

Better health and renewed energy counts affect the appearance of the skin. You should see improvements in blood sugar and lipid levels and cardiovascular safety. You will experience better levels of triglycerides and cholesterol.

Losing weight aside, incorporating sirtfoods into your diet is a big step towards making your cells more disease-resistant, setting you up for a longer lifespan.

HOW TO FOLLOW PHASE 1

In order to make Phase 1 smooth sailing, we will lead you one day at a time through the whole seven-day cycle, along with a full rundown on the sirtfood green smoothie and easy-to-follow, tasty meals.

Stage 1 of the Sirtfood Diet:

Days 1 to 3 are the most intense, and you can consume up to thousand calories per day during this time, comprised of:

- 3 x sirtfood green vegetable juices
- 1 x main diet

Days 4 to 7: You see your caloric intake rise to a daily limit of fifteen hundred calories, composed of:

- 2 x sirtfood green vegetable juices
- 2 x main diets

There are few rules to obey the diet. Undoubtedly, for sustained progress, it's about incorporating the diet into your daily life. Here are a recommendations for best results:

1: Get a good juicer: fruit juice is an essential part of sirtfood nutrition, and a blender is one of the important purchases you'll make. While expenditure is key, some mixers are more efficient at extracting the juice from leafy greens vegetables and herbs.

2: Preparation Is key: from feedback, we know that those who scheduled ahead of time were the most successful. Get to know the required food ingredients and methods, and start stocking up. You'd be surprised at how easy the entire process is with almost everything coordinated and prepared.

3. Save time: If time is tight, get clever. Food should be prepared the previous night. Liquids can be made in quantity and stored in the refrigerator for up to 3 days (or further in the freezer) until their sirtuin-activating nutrient uptake begin to decrease. Shield it from sunlight.

4. Eat early: Eating fairly early in the day is nice and preferable. Food and juices should not be ingested later than 7 p.m. The diet is essentially tailored for this routine, but late people who eat can still profit.

5. Space out the juices: To increase the uptake of green juices, they must be ingested at least 1 hour before or 2 hours after a meal and distributed throughout the day, instead of being close to each other.

6. Eat until satisfied: Sirtfoods may have a serious impact on hunger, and some people will be exhausted until their diet is over. Pay attention to your body and eat till fulfilled, rather than shoving down the food. Say, "Hara hachi bu," as the long-living Okinawans do, which translates literally as, "Eat until you are eighty percent jampacked."

7. Enjoy the journey: don't obsess on the ultimate objective; instead, process the adventure with joy. This diet is about commemorating food in all its mystery, for its beneficial effects, but also for the pleasure and satisfaction it brings. Studies suggest that we are much more likely to be successful if we keep our eyes concentrated on the road rather than the ultimate goal.

What to Drink

The required daily quantities of green juices and other drinks should be heeded in Phase 1 - non-calorie beverages, ideally plain juice, black coffee, and herbal tea. If your standard preference is for dark or herbal teas, do not hesitate to include these. Fruit juices and carbonated beverages are to be left behind. Rather, consider adding a few sliced strawberries to sparkling water to make your own sirtfood-infused health cocktail if you'd like to spice things up. Keep it for a few hours in the fridge and you will have a delightful and fascinating substitute for sugary soft drinks and juices.

One thing you need to be conscious of is that we don't advise sudden major changes to your standard coffee use.

Caffeine's side effects may make you feel shockingly bad for a few days. Similarly, large quantities may be awkward for those especially sensitive to the impact of caffeine. We suggest drinking coffee black without milk, as some studies have found that adding milk minimizes the absorption of the important nutrients that trigger sirtuin. The same was found for green tea, although adding some lemon juice definitely improves the strength of the nutrients that activate sirtuin.

Realize that this is the phase of high energy-success, and while you are comforted by the reality that this is only for a whole week, you have to be conscientious. We usually add alcohol for last week in the form of red wine as a food preservative.

THE SIRTFOOD GREEN JUICE

Green juice is an important component of the Sirtfood Diet's Phase 1 program. All the components are strong sirtfoods, and with each juice you get the great advantage of natural products like apigenin, kaempferol, luteolin, quercetin, and EGCG that function together in turning on the sirtuin genes and encourage fat burning. We add lemon as its inherent acidity has been shown to secure, maintain and improve the ingestion of the sirtuin-activating components of the drink. We have added a bit of apple and ginger for flavor, too. All are readily available.

SIRTFOOD GREEN JUICE (SERVES 1)

1. 2 large handfuls (about 2 1 /2 ounces or 75g) kale

2. a large handful (1 ounce or 30g) arugula

3. a very small handful (about 1 /4 ounce or 5g) at-leaf parsley

4. 2 to 3 large celery stalks (5 1 /2 ounces or 150g), including leaves

5. 1 /2 medium green apple

6. 1 /2- to 1-inch (1 to 2.5 cm) piece of fresh ginger

7. juice of 1 /2 lemon

8. 1 /2 level teaspoon matcha powder

Days 1 to 3 of Phase 1: add only to the first two juices of the day.

Days 4 to 7 of Phase 1: add to both juices

We balance the amounts per our study, tailoring the quantity of nutrients to the body size of an ordinary person. Larger people get a substantially greater amount of sirtfood nutrients to meet their physical attributes.

- Mix the greens together (kale, arugula, and parsley) and sauté them. Mixers vary in their effectiveness when juicing leafy green vegetables. The target is to end up with about 2 pounds of liquid or near to 1/4 cup (50ml) of green vegetable juice.

- Now juice the apple, celery, and ginger juice.

- Slice the lemon and place it in the blender. We find it easier to push juice the lemon by hand. You get approximately 1 cup (250ml) of juice in maximum, maybe more.
- You add matcha. In a bowl, place a small amount of water then add the matcha and mix rapidly with a fork. For the first two cups of the day, we only use matcha, as it has levels of caffeine (the same quality as a regular cup of tea). If consumed late, it will keep you up at night.
- Add any remaining juice once the matcha is integrated. Give it a swirl. Top it off with simple tea if you want.

PHASE 1: YOUR SEVEN-DAY GUIDE

And now the benefit begins. Drink the juice at various times during twenty four hours for days 1 to 3 (e.g. the very first thing every morning, mid-morning and late-afternoon) and choose one of the regular or vegetarian meal choices we offer. Consume them at a time and place of choice (generally dinner or lunch).

Day 1

On Day 1, you will consume

- 3 x Sirtfood green juices
- 1 x main meal (standard or vegan option), either

Asian shrimp stir-fry with buckwheat noodles

+

1 /2 to 3 /4 ounce (15 to 20g) dark chocolate (85 percent cocoa solids)

or

Miso and sesame glazed tofu with ginger and chili stir-fried greens (vegan)

+

1 /2 to 3 /4 ounce (15 to 20g) dark chocolate (85 percent cocoa solids)

Day 2

On Day 2, you will consume

- 3 x sirtfood green juices
- 1 x main meal (standard or vegan option), either

Turkey escalope with sage, capers, and parsley and spiced cauliflower "couscous"

+

1 /2 to 3 /4 ounce (15 to 20g) dark chocolate (85 percent cocoa solids)

or

Kale and red onion dal with buckwheat (vegan)

+

1 /2 to 3 /4 ounce (15 to 20g) dark chocolate (85 percent cocoa solids)

Day 3

On Day 3, you will consume

- 3 x sirtfood green juices
- 1 x main meal (standard or vegan option), either

Aromatic chicken breast with kale and red onions and a tomato and chili salsa

+

1 /2 to 3 /4 ounce (15 to 20g) dark chocolate (85 percent cocoa solids)

or

Harissa baked tofu with cauliflower "couscous" (vegan)

+

1 /2 to 3 /4 ounce (15 to 20g) dark chocolate (85 percent cocoa solids)

Start drinking the juice at different times of the day for days four to seven (e.g. either in the morning or late morning with the second in the late afternoon). Then choose your meals from either our conventional or vegetarian cuisine and consume them at the right time (usually ingested for breakfast, dinner and lunch). You may add dark chocolate (eighty five percent cocoa solids) in 1/2 to 3/4 ounces (15 to 20 g) every day, depending on your preference.

Day 4

On Day 4, you will consume

- 2 x sirtfood green juices
- 2 x main meals (standard or vegan option), either

MEAL 1: Sirt muesli

MEAL 2: Pan-fried salmon fillet with caramelized endive, arugula, and celery leaf salad

or

MEAL 1: Sirt muesli (vegan)

MEAL 2: Tuscan bean stew (vegan)

Day 5

On Day 5, you will consume

• 2 x sirtfood green juices

• 2 x main meals (standard or vegan option), either

MEAL 1: Strawberry buckwheat tabbouleh

MEAL 2: Miso-marinated baked cod with stir-fried greens and

sesame

or

MEAL 1: Strawberry buckwheat tabbouleh (vegan)

MEAL 2: Soba (buckwheat noodles) in a miso broth with tofu, celery, and kale (vegan)

Day 6

On Day 6, you will consume

- 2 x sirtfood green juices
- 2 x main meals (standard or vegan option), either

MEAL 1: Sirt super salad

MEAL 2: Char-grilled beef with a red wine jus, onion rings, garlic kale, and herb-roasted potatoes

or

MEAL 1: Lentil sirt super salad (vegan)

MEAL 2: Kidney bean mole with baked potato (vegan)

Day 7

On Day 7, you will consume

- 2 x sirtfood green juices
- 2 x main meals (standard or vegan option), either

MEAL 1: Sirtfood omelet

MEAL 2: Baked chicken breast with walnut and parsley pesto and red onion salad

or

MEAL 1: Waldorf salad (vegan)

MEAL 2: Roasted eggplant wedges with walnut and parsley pesto and tomato salad (vegan)

PHASE 2: MAINTENANCE

Kudos on finishing Sirtfood Diet step 1! You will now see amazing progress and a weight reduction. You not only look thinner and more muscular but also feel transformed and re-energized. So, what's next?

While everyone else has seen these always-remarkable modifications, we know you want to see even greater outcomes, not just the maintenance all the acquired advantages. Sirtfoods are, after all, meant to be eaten for life. The issue is how you customize what you did in Phase 1 into your daily nutritional routine. This is precisely what inspired us to develop a 14-day maintenance schedule to help you make the shift from Phase 1 to a daily nutritional regimen, thus helping you maintain and expand the advantages of the Sirtfood Diet.

WHAT TO EXPECT

You will maintain the weight loss results through Step 2 and start to lose weight gradually.

The one surprising point we've seen with the Sirtfood Diet is that much or all obese people lose fat, and many definitely acquire strength. Therefore, we would like to remind you that you shouldn't just evaluate your success by measurements alone. Look in a mirror to see if you look thinner and more muscular; see how well your clothes fits, and gobble up the nice comments you'll get.

Also remember that as the weight loss continues, so will the medical benefits. By following our 14-day maintenance program, you are indeed beginning to lay the groundwork for long-term health.

HOW TO FOLLOW PHASE 2

The trick to progress now is having your nutrition packed full of sirtfoods. To render it as simple as possible, we have prepared a seven-day meal schedule to fulfill the requirements. Our tasty and healthy recipes are filled with sirtfoods to the rafters. All you have to do is replicate the Seven Day Schedule again to fulfill the 14 days of Step 2.

On each of the fourteen days your diet will consist of

- 3 x balanced sirtfood-enriched meals
- 1 x sirtfood green vegetable juice
- 1 to 2 x optional sirtfood bite snacks

There are no strict rules. Be flexible throughout the day and follow them. Two basic rules of thumb are:

- Have your green vegetable juice either early in the morning, at least thirty minutes before breakfast, or in the middle of the morning.
- Do your best to finish your dinner before 7 p.m.

PORTION SIZES

In the second phase, attention is not on counting calories. For the average person, it is not a realistic solution or even an effective one. Rather we concentrate on healthy servings, well-balanced meals and, most importantly, loading up on sirtfoods so you can start to profit from their gat-burning and health impact.

We have a strategy to make you feel full and satisfied. Synchronized with sirtfoods' natural hunger-regulating effects, you're not going to spend the next 14 days feeling hungry, but satisfied, well-fed, and well-nourished.

Just like in Phase 1, listen attentively and be directed by your desire to eat. When you prepare food as per our directions and consider that you will be full before you have completed a meal, ceasing to eat is completely acceptable!

WHAT TO DRINK

Through most of Step 2, you'll have one green vegetable juice daily. This is to maintain your high sirtfoods level. As in Phase 1, you can easily imbibe certain fluids in Phase 2. Our favorite beverages comprise plain beer, bottled sweet soda, coffee, and green tea. If black or white tea is your predisposition, please enjoy. The very same holds for black tea. The biggest issue is that throughout Phase 2 you can enjoy an occasional glass of red wine. Due to its high content of sirtuin-activating polyphenols, particularly resveratrol and piceatannol, red wine is a sirtfood that is by far the best alcoholic drink. As liquor causes a negative impact on tissue, restraint is always safest, and we suggest restricting yourself to one glass of red wine with food for 2 to 3 days a week during Phase 2.

RETURNING TO THREE MEALS

You ingested only one or two meals per day during Phase 1 which allowed you plenty of flexibility. Since we are returning to our usual schedule and the well-tested practice of 3 meals a day, learning about breakfast is a timely idea.

Eating a nutritious breakfast sets us up for the day, raising our energy and focus. Eating early keeps our blood glucose and fat levels in balance, in terms of metabolism. That this meal is beneficial is pointed out by a series of studies that find that individuals who eat breakfast are less probable to obesity.

This is because of our body's internal rhythms. Our organs are asking us to eat early in expectation of when we will be busier and need food. Yet more than a third of us will miss breakfast on any given day. It's a typical example of our crazy daily lives where there's just not enough time to eat properly. But as you can see, nothing could be farther from the truth. So we have great options. Whether it's the sirtfood smoothie to drink on the go, the premade sirt muesli, or the fast and simple sirtfood scrambled eggs/tofu, taking a bit of time will yield rewards not only for your whole day but also for your fitness and wellbeing long term.

With sirtfoods' ability to surcharge our metabolism, we get a boost from them early in the morning. It is done not only by eating a sirtfood-rich meal, but by consuming the green vegetable juice either first thing every morning — at least 30 minutes before meal — or late-morning. We hear a lot of stories about people who first sip their green vegetable juice and don't feel thirsty for a few hours afterwards. If that is the impact it has on you, waiting a few hours before eating breakfast is fine. Just don't miss this one. Conversely, with a healthy meal starting your day, wait for two or three hours to have the green vegetable juice. Go with anything that appeals to you.

SIRTFOOD BITES

Eat it or leave it. There has been much discussion on whether eating regular, smaller meals is better for losing weight, or only sticking to 3 healthy meals a day. The reality is that it is not really relevant.

The way we've built the servicing menu guarantees you 're going to eat 3 well-balanced sirtfood-rich meals a day; and you might find that you don't always need a snack. So maybe you've been engaged with the kids in the classroom, going out or dashing about, and need something to last you until the next meal. But if that "little thing" offers you a whammy of sirtfood vitamins and minerals along with a wonderful taste, then it's a good time to dig in. Thus we developed our "Sirtfood Bits." These fun little treats are a truly misery-free choice made completely from sirtfoods: almonds, walnuts, chocolate, turmeric, and extra virgin olive oil. We suggest eating one, or possibly two, every other day on days when you really need them.

"SIRTIFYING" YOUR MEALS

We have found that the only consistent meals are those of acceptance, not removal. Yet real achievement goes well beyond that — the diet needs to be consistent with modern life. If about the ease of satisfying the needs of our stressful lifestyle or keeping with our role at social events as the bon vivant. In any case, the way we eat should be trouble-free. You will admire your svelte body and beautiful smile, rather than thinking about the requirements and limitations of kooky products.

What makes sirtfoods so fabulous is that they are readily available, common, and simple to include in your eating habits. When you cross the distance between step 1 and daily eating, you lay the groundwork for a new, enhanced lifelong nutrition strategy.

The basic feature of your meal options is "sirtifying." This is where we take popular meals, along with several classic favorites, and we retain all the fantastic flavor with some smart swaps and easy sirtfood additions. You'll see how conveniently this is accomplished across Phase 2.

Highlights include our tasty smoothie sirtfood for the ultimate on-the-go breakfast in a time-consuming universe, and the easy turn from wheat to buckwheat to bring more flavor and bite to a much-loved pasta meal. In the meantime, famous, adored meals such as chili con carne and curry won't even need a transition, with sirtfood bonanzas imbuing local dishes.

So, who says that junk food means bad food? When you start making it yourself, we integrate the lively ingredients of a pizza without the culpability. There's no reason to say goodbye to pleasures either, as our pancakes with fruit and dark chocolate pudding demonstrate. It's not just cake, it's breakfast and for you and it's perfect. Easy shift: you keep eating the food you enjoy while maintaining a good weight and stability. This is the Sirtfood diet movement.

COOKING FOR MORE

We accept that we are undergoing a time of "sirtfoods for everyone," where meals appeal to many more mouths. If it's for friends or family members. The latest suppers as well as our sirtfood-packed soup are planned with everyone in mind. Why not reap the benefits of preparing a batch of food to freeze rather than cooking every day?

FOURTEEN-DAY MEAL PLAN

Besides our pro package, we also have a meat-free edition fit for vegetarians. Experiment and pick with whatever you want.

Each day you will consume

- 1 x sirtfood green juice
- 3 x main meals (standard or vegan options,)
- 1 to 2 x optional sirtfood bites

Drink the juice whether in the morning, at least 30 minutes before breakfast, or in the late morning.

BREAKFAST

Day 8 and 15

- Sirtfood smoothie

Day 9 and 16

- Sirt muesli

Day 10 and 17

- Yogurt with mixed berries, chopped walnuts, and dark chocolate

or

- Soy or coconut yogurt with mixed berries, chopped walnuts, and dark chocolate

Day 11 and 18

- Spiced scrambled eggs

or

- Mushroom and tofu scramble

Day 12 and 19

- Sirtfood smoothie

Day 13 and 20

- Buckwheat pancakes with strawberries, chocolate sauce, and crushed walnuts

or

- Soy or coconut yogurt with mixed berries, chopped walnuts, and dark chocolate

Day 14 and 21

- Sirtfood omelet

or

- Sirt muesli

LUNCH	DINNER
Chicken Sirt super salad	Asian shrimp stir-fry with buckwheat noodles
Waldorf salad	Tuscan bean stew
Stuffed whole-wheat pita	Butternut squash and date tagine with buckwheat
Butter bean and miso dip with celery sticks and oatcakes	Butternut squash and date tagine with buckwheat
Tuna Sirt super salad	Chicken and kale curry with Bombay potatoes
Stuffed whole-wheat pita	Kale and red onion dal with buckwheat
Strawberry buckwheat tabbouleh	Sirt chili con carne
Strawberry buckwheat tabbouleh*	Kidney bean mole with baked potato*
Waldorf salad	Smoked salmon pasta with chili and arugula
Buckwheat pasta salad	Harissa baked tofu with cauliflower "couscous"

Tofu and shiitake mushroom soup	Sirtfood pizza
Tofu and shiitake mushroom soup	Sirtfood pizza
Lentil Sirt super salad	Baked chicken breast with walnut and parsley pesto and red onion salad
Lentil Sirt super salad	Miso and sesame glazed tofu with ginger and chili stir-fried greens

After the Diet

Congrats, all Sirtfood Diet phases have now ceased! Let's take stock of what you've achieved. You have reached the hyper-success point, experiencing weight loss in the realm of 7 pounds, which may involve some attractive muscle development. During the fourteen-day maintenance process, you maintained your weight loss and further improved your body composition. Above all, you've marked the beginning of your own personal health revolution. You have taken a stand against the tide of ill health which strikes as we age. The future you have chosen is full of greater energy, resilience, and wellbeing.

We've seen why sirtfoods are so advantageous: some plants have intricate stress-response mechanisms that generate compounds that further activate sirtuins — the same fat-burning and longevity mechanism triggered by fasting and exercise. The larger the quantity of the compounds that plants produce in response to stress, the greater the value we derive from eating them. The best twenty sirtfoods consist of foods that really stand out since they are particularly packed full of these compounds. Therefore, they are the foods with the most extraordinary ability to impact the composition and well-being of the body.

But the sirtuin-activating effects of foods aren't a whole or nothing concept. There are many other crops out there that contain moderate amounts of sirtuin-activating antioxidants. We allow you to further increase the range and diversity of your diet by consuming them liberally. The Sirtfood Diet is all about inclusion; the greater the range of sirtuin activating foods that can be added to the diet, the better the results. Particularly if it means reaping more from your favorite foods to maximize enjoyment and pleasure.

These two stages can be reworked as often as you like to for additional weight reduction. Be that as it may, you are urged to keep eating the sirtifying regimen after these stages have been completed, by consistently consolidating sirt foods into your meals.

There are all kinds of Sirtfood Diet books filled with sirtfood-rich plans. You can also incorporate sirtfoods as tidbits into your eating routine or use them according to plan plans. You're encouraged to continue drinking the green juice every day.

The Sirtfood Diet thus turns out to be a way of life that changes users to a greater extent than a single diet.

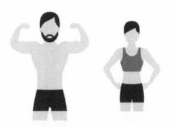

Chapter 6:

How to Lose Fat

LIST OF SIRTUIN ACTIVATING, FAT BURNING SIRT FOODS

Sirt foods contain naturally occurring compounds that are known to activate sirtuin proteins. These sirtuin activators include powerful antioxidants called polyphenols.

Almond	Apple cider vinegar	Apples
Apricots	Asparagus	Aubergine/eggplant
Avocado	Balsamic vinegar	Bananas
Bean sprouts	Bell peppers	Blackcurrants
Black garlic	Black grapes	Blueberries
Brazil nuts	Broccoli	Buckwheat
Cabbages	Capers	Carrot
Cauliflower	Celeriac	Celery
Cherries	Chia seeds	Chickpeas (garbanzo beans)
Chicory	Chillies	Cocoa
Coconut	Coffee	Corn
Cranberries	Dark chocolate	Dates
Eggs	Elderberries	Fava (broad) beans
Fennel	Figs	Flaxseed
Garlic	Globe artichokes	Goji berries
Gooseberries	Grapefruit	Guava
Hazelnuts	Horseradish	Kale
Kidney beans	Lemons	Lentils
Lettuce	Limes	Macadamia nuts
Mango	Mangosteen	Miso soup
Mushrooms	Oily fish	Olives
Olive oil	Onions	Oranges

Pak choi / bok choy	Papaya	Passion fruit
Peanuts	Pears	Pecans
Physalis (Cape gooseberry)	Pine nuts	Pineapple
Pistachios	Plums	Pomegranate
Prunes	Pumpkin	Pumpkin seeds
Purple Potato	Red Grapes	Red kidney beans
Red onions	Rocket (arugula)	Rye
Soybeans	Spinach	Strawberries
Sweetcorn	Sweet potato	Tomatoes
Walnuts	Watercress	Watermelon

Herbs and spices

Most herbs and spices are powerful sirtuin activators, including clove, black pepper, cinnamon, cardamom, cumin, coriander, lemon verbena, mint, ginger, oregano, nutmeg, rosemary, parsley, thyme, sage, turmeric, and edible flowers.

Fat burning drinks

Green tea, black tea, white tea, matcha, chamomile tea, rooibos and red wine (one glass per day).

If you eat nothing but the above foods, you will definitely lose weight!

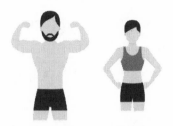

Chapter 7:
Sirtfood Recipes

Some important notes concerning these recipes:

1. The recipes mention Thai chilies (also known as chilies with bird's eye). They are notably hotter than regular chilies if you've never had them before. If you are not used to spicy cooking, we recommend you begin with a milder chili such as serrano, and change the amount to suit your taste. Once you get more used to having chilies daily in your diet, you may notice that you are beginning to love the hotter varieties, so please do try them.

2. Miso is a tasty fermented soybean paste, loaded with flavor. It comes in a variety of colors, usually white, yellow, red, and brown. The sweeter miso pastes are lighter in color than the dark ones, which can be very salty. Brown or red miso should serve well for our recipes, so play with it by all means to see which taste you like. Red miso seems to be the saltier version, so you may choose to use a little less if you go for this one. Miso's flavor and saltiness can also vary from product to product, so the best option would be to verify which kinds to buy and change the amount you use appropriately, so it isn't too intoxicating. This requires a bit of trial and error, but eventually you'll get the best of it.

3. It couldn't be better if you haven't eaten buckwheat yet. We suggest you rinse the buckwheat vigorously in a sieve first before putting it in a saucepan of hot water. Baking times can vary so verify the guidelines.

4. It would be better for all meals to have flat-leaf parsley, but if you can't get it, frizzy will do.

5. Onions, garlic, and ginger should always be removed unless stated otherwise.

6. These recipes do not use salt and pepper, but feel free to season with sea salt and black pepper to suit your own personal tastes. Sirtfoods deliver so much flavor

that you'll actually find that you don't need as many seasonings as usually. It is strongly suggested to add black pepper to any dish that includes turmeric, because this will further improve the absorption of the main sirtuin-activating compound, curcumin.

Metric Conversion Chart

Grams(g)	Ounces(oz)	Grams(g)	Ounces(oz)
0 g	0 oz	7 g	0.2469 oz
1 g	0.0353 oz	8 g	0.2822 oz
2 g	0.0706 oz	9 g	0.3175 oz
3 g	0.1058 oz	10 g	0.3527 oz
4 g	0.1411 oz	20 g	0.7055 oz
5 g	0.1764 oz	30 g	1.0582 oz
6 g	0.2116 oz	40 g	1.4110 oz

To convert grams to ounces, multiply **grams x 0.03527396195 oz.**

ASIAN SHRIMP STIR-FRY WITH
BUCKWHEAT NOODLES

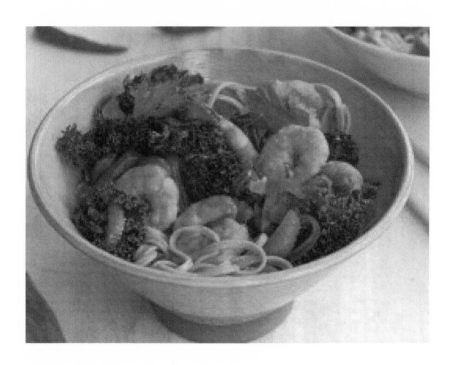

Ingredients	Quantity
shelled raw jumbo shrimp, deveined	1/3 pound (150g)
tamari (or soy sauce if not avoiding gluten)	2 teaspoons
extra virgin olive oil	2 teaspoons
soba (buckwheat noodles)	3 ounces (75g)
garlic cloves, finely sliced	2

Thai chili, finely sliced	1
teaspoon finely sliced fresh ginger	1
red onions, sliced	1/8 cup (20g)
celery including leaves, trimmed, and sliced, with leaves set aside	1/2 cup (45g)
green beans, chopped	1/2 cup (75g)
kale, roughly chopped	3/4 cup (50g)
chicken stock	1/2 cup (100ml)

Serves 1

INSTRUCTIONS

1. Put a deep fryer on a high temperature, then cook the shrimp for two or three minutes in 1 tablespoon tamari and one teaspoon oil. Put the shrimp on a tray. Wipe the skillet down with a paper towel, as you will be using it again.

2. Bake the noodles for five to eight minutes in boiling water, or as indicated on the box. Drain and set aside.

3. In the leftover tamari and oil over medium-high heat, cook the garlic, ginger, chili, celery (but not the leaves), red onion, kale and green beans for two to three

minutes. Bring the stock to a simmer for a couple of minutes until the vegetables are done yet crunchy.

4. Add the shrimp, pasta, and celery foliage to a bowl, bring to a simmer again, turn off the heat and enjoy.

MISO AND SESAME GLAZED TOFU WITH GINGER AND CHILI STIR-FRIED GREENS

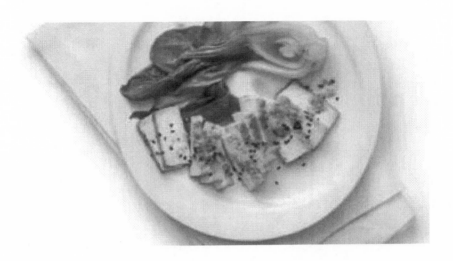

Ingredients	Quantity
Mirin	1 tablespoon
miso paste	3 ¹/² teaspoons (20g)
block of rm tofu	1 x 5-ounce (150g)
celery, trimmed (about 1/3 cup sliced)	1 stalk (40g)
red onion, sliced	1/4 cup (40g)
zucchini (about 1 cup sliced)	1 small (120g)
Thai chili	1
garlic cloves	2
teaspoon finely sliced fresh ginger	1

kale, chopped	3 /4 cup (50g)
sesame seeds	2 teaspoons
Buckwheat	1 /4 cup (35g)
ground turmeric	1 teaspoon
extra virgin olive oil	2 teaspoons
tamari (or soy sauce if not avoiding gluten)	1 teaspoon

Serves 1

INSTRUCTIONS

1. Heat oven to 400oF (200oC). Line a baking dish with thin parchment paper.
2. Blend both the mirin and the miso. Cut tofu lengthwise, then in a diagonal direction split each slice into a triangle. Wrap the tofu with the miso mixture and allow to marinate while the other items are prepared.
3. Chop the celery and red onion. Chop the chili, garlic, and ginger thinly, and set aside.
4. Heat the kale for five minutes in a container. Set aside.
5. Put the tofu in a baking dish, stir in sesame seeds and bake in the oven for fifteen to twenty minutes until beautifully caramelized.
6. Strain the buckwheat with mesh, then put along with the turmeric in a saucepan of boiling hot water. Process

as indicated on the box then rinse. Heat the oil in a saucepan and add the onion, celery, zucchini, chili, garlic, and ginger.

7. Fry over high heat for one to two minutes, then decrease to a moderate flame for approximately 3 minutes until the vegetables are cooked through yet crunchy. If the vegetables start sticking to the skillet, you may have to add a spoonful of water. Add the tamari and kale and cook for 1 minute.

8. Top with the leaves and buckwheat after the tofu has set.

TURKEY ESCALOPE WITH SAGE, CAPERS, AND PARSLEY AND SPICED CAULIFLOWER "COUSCOUS"

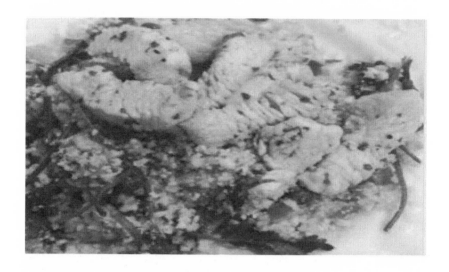

Slender cutlets are great but there are two good ways to turn them into an escalope when using turkey breasts. You should either use a meat tenderizer, a spike, or a rolling pin to tenderize the poultry pieces until they are around 1/4 inch (5 mm) thick, based on how dense the meat is. Alternatively, if you find the breasts are too hard to deal with and you have a strong hand, split the chest in half horizontally and tenderize.

Ingredients	Quantity
cauliflower, roughly chopped	1 1/2 cups (150g)
garlic cloves, finely sliced	2
red onion, finely sliced	1/4 cup (40g)
Thai chili, finely sliced	1
finely sliced fresh ginger	1 teaspoon
extra virgin olive oil	2 tablespoons
ground turmeric	2 teaspoons
sun-dried tomatoes, finely sliced	1/2 cup (30g)
fresh parsley, chopped	1/4 cup (10g)
turkey cutlet or steak (see above)	1/3-pound (150g)
dried sage	1 teaspoon
juice of lemon	1/4
Capers	1 tablespoon

Serves 1

INSTRUCTIONS

1. Put the raw cabbage in a mixing bowl to produce the "couscous." Finely slice the cabbage with a knife or food processor.

2. In 1 tablespoon of the oil, cook the red onion, garlic, chili, and ginger until soft but not browned. Add in the cabbage and turmeric and continue cooking for one minute. Remove the tomatoes from pan and add half of the parsley.

3. Cover the escalope with the herbs and just a little butter, then cook in a large skillet over medium heat for four to six minutes using the residual oil and turning periodically. Add the lemon juice, remaining parsley, capers and 1 tablespoon of water to the skillet to make a cabbage sauce.

KALE AND RED ONION DAL
WITH BUCKWHEAT

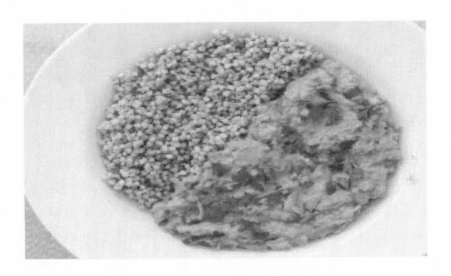

Ingredients	Quantity
extra virgin olive oil	1 teaspoon
mustard seeds	1 teaspoon
red onion, finely sliced	1/4 cup (40g)
garlic cloves, finely sliced	2
finely sliced fresh ginger	1 teaspoon
Thai chili, finely sliced	1
mild curry powder (medium or hot as you prefer)	1 teaspoon
ground turmeric	2 teaspoons
vegetable stock or water	1 1/4 cups (300ml)

red lentils, rinsed	1/4 cup (40g)
kale, chopped	3/4 cup (50g)
tinned coconut milk	3 1/2 tablespoons (50ml)
buckwheat	1/3 cup (50g)

Serves 1

INSTRUCTIONS

1. Heat the oil over moderate heat in a small saucepan and add the mustard seeds. When the mustard seeds begin popping, introduce the onion, ginger, garlic, and chili. Fry until smooth, for about ten minutes.

2. Add one tablespoon of turmeric curry powder and steam the seasoning for a few minutes. Stir the stock and bring to a simmer. Attach the lentils to the saucepan and boil for another twenty-five to thirty minutes until the lentils are fried, producing a glossy dal is available.

3. Start adding milk to the kale and coconut and bake for another five minutes.

4. In the meantime, fry the buckwheat with the leftover turmeric tablespoon, as per the box instructions. Drain and eat with the dal.

AROMATIC CHICKEN BREAST WITH KALE AND RED ONIONS AND A TOMATO AND CHILI SALSA

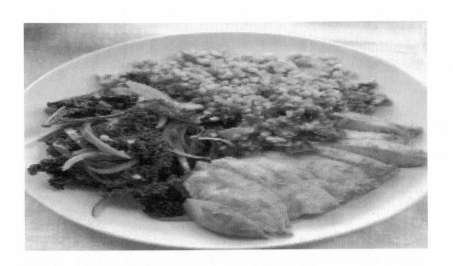

Ingredients	Quantity
skinless, boneless chicken breast	1/4 pound (120g)
ground turmeric	2 teaspoons
juice of lemon	¼
extra-virgin olive oil	1 tablespoon
kale, chopped	3/4 cup (50g)
red onion, sliced	1/8 cup (20g)
chopped fresh ginger	1 teaspoon
Buckwheat	1/3 cup (50g)

FOR THE SALSA

medium tomato	1 of (130g)
Thai chili, finely sliced	1
capers, finely sliced	1 tablespoon
parsley, finely sliced	2 tablespoons (5g)
juice of lemon	¼
Serves 1	

INSTRUCTIONS

1. Start by removing the stem from the tomato to make the salsa and slice it well, taking care to keep as much of the fluid as possible. Blend with the chili, parsley, capers, and lemon juice. You can put it all in a mixer, but the final outcome is a little different.

2. Heat the oven to 220 ° C (4250F). In one teaspoon of turmeric, the lemon juice, and a little oil, bake the roast chicken for five to ten minutes.

3. Heat an oven-proof deep fryer until warm, then introduce the marinated chicken and roast on each side for a moment or until a pale golden color, then switch to the oven (set on a cookie sheet if your skillet is not oven-proof) for eight to ten minutes or till roasted. Remove from heat, wrap in foil, then leave for five minutes before having to serve.

4. In the meantime, boil the kale for five minutes in a container. Cook the red onions and ginger in a little oil, then add the cooked kale and cook till smooth but not golden brown.

5. Fry the buckwheat with the residual turmeric tablespoon, as per the package directions. Serve with the meat, leafy greens, and salsa.

HARISSA BAKED TOFU WITH CAULIFLOWER "COUSCOUS"

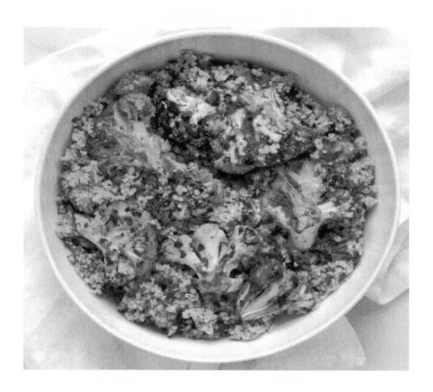

Ingredients	Quantity
red bell pepper	3/8 cup (60g)
Thai chili, cut in half	1
garlic cloves	2
extra-virgin olive oil	about 1 tablespoon
ground cumin	pinch of
ground coriander	pinch of

juice of lemon	¼
rm tofu	7 ounces (200g)
cauliflower, roughly chopped	1 3/4 cups (200g)
red onion, finely sliced	1/4 cup (40g)
finely sliced fresh ginger	1 teaspoon
ground turmeric	2 teaspoons
sun-dried tomatoes, finely sliced	1/2 cup (30g)
parsley, chopped	1/2 cup (20g)

Serves 1

INSTRUCTIONS

1. Heat the oven to 400°F (200°C).

2. Chop the long red pepper in the center to make the harissa so you have good-sized pieces and remove any seeds, after which place the chili and one of the garlic cloves in a baking dish. Add a little oil and the thawed cumin and coriander and bake for fifteen to twenty minutes till the peppers are smooth but not gray. (Leave the oven at this setting.) Then mix with the lemon juice in a mixing bowl till light and fluffy.

3. Make chunks with the tofu then in the diagonal direction cut each into triangles. In a small detachable casserole dish or one lined with baking parchment,

place the harissa and grill for twenty minutes in the oven — the tofu should consume the marinade and started turning dark red.

4. To make the "couscous," cut the raw cauliflower in meal.

5. Thinly slice and dice the cabbage till it mimics couscous.

6. Open the last clove of garlic. In one tablespoon of oil, roast the ginger, red onion, and garlic until softened but not golden brown, then introduce the turmeric and cabbage and cook over medium heat for one minute.

7. Remove from heat and mix in the tomatoes and parsley. Serve with the fried tofu.

SIRT MUESLI

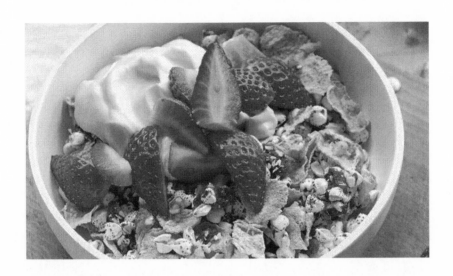

Combine the dry ingredients and put the combination in an enclosed jar if you want to make a large quantity or cook it the evening before. The very next day all you have to do is introduce the strawberries and milk, and it's ready to go.

Ingredients	Quantity
buckwheat flakes	1/4 cup (20g)
buckwheat puffs	2/3 cup (10g)
coconut flakes or dried coconut	3 tablespoons (15g)
Medjool dates, pitted and chopped	1/4 cup (40g)
walnuts, chopped	1/8 cup (15g)

cocoa nibs	1 1/2 tablespoons (10g)
strawberries, hulled and chopped	2/3 cup (100g)
plain Greek yogurt (or vegan alternative, such as soy or coconut yogurt)	3/8 cup (100g)

Serves 1

INSTRUCTIONS

1. Mix all the ingredients together (leave out the strawberries and yogurt if not serving right away).

PAN-FRIED SALMON FILLET WITH CARAMELIZED ENDIVE, ARUGULA, AND CELERY LEAF SALAD

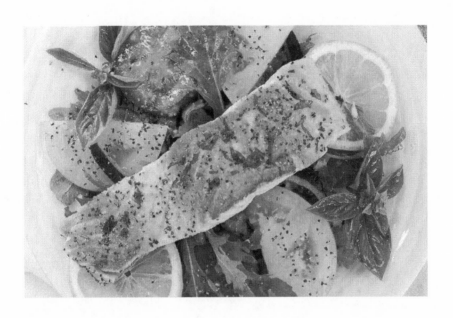

Ingredients	Quantity
Parsley	1/4 cup (10g)
juice of lemon	¼
capers	1 tablespoon
clove garlic, roughly chopped	1
extra-virgin olive oil	1 tablespoon
avocado, peeled, stoned, and diced	1/4

cherry tomatoes, cut in half	2/3 cup (100g)
red onion, thinly sliced	1/8 cup (20g)
arugula	1 3/4 ounces (50g)
celery leaves	2 tablespoons (5g)
skinless salmon fillet	1 x 5-ounce (150g)
brown sugar	2 teaspoons
head of endive (1), cut in half *lengthways*	about 2 1/2 ounces (70g)

Serves 1

INSTRUCTIONS

1. Heat the oven to 220 ° C (4250F).

2. Put the parsley, garlic, lemon juice, capers, and two teaspoons of oil in a mixing bowl or blender for the dressing and mix until thick and creamy.

3. For the salad, combine the leaves of a red onion, the tomato, arugula, avocado and celery.

4. Heat a frying pan over a high temperature. Massage the salmon in a little oil and sear for a moment in the skillet to caramelize the exterior. Transfer to a small bowl and bake in the oven for four to six minutes or until it has finished cooking.

5. Decrease the heating process by two minutes if you like your fish pink on the inside.

6. Wash the pan out and put everything back on high heat. Mix the brown sugar with the remaining oil teaspoon and sprinkle over cut endive. Place the endive in the skillet and cook for two or three minutes, turning frequently until tender and perfectly golden brown.

7. Mix the salad and top with the salmon and endive.

TUSCAN BEAN STEW

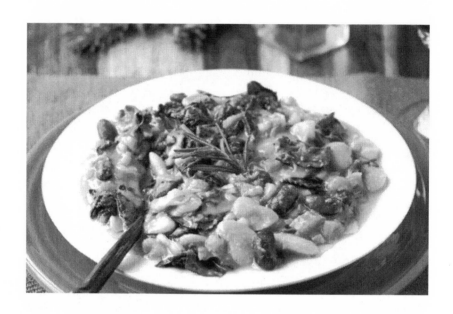

Ingredients	Quantity
extra-virgin olive oil	1 tablespoon
red onion, finely chopped	1/3 cup (50g)
carrot, peeled and finely sliced	1/4 cup (30g)
celery, trimmed and finely sliced	1/3 cup (30g)
garlic cloves, finely sliced	2
Thai chili, finely sliced (optional)	1/2
herbs de Provence	1 teaspoon

vegetable stock	7/8 cup (200ml)
chopped Italian tomatoes	1 x 14-ounce can (400g)
tomato purée	1 teaspoon
canned mixed beans (drained weight)	3/4 cup (130g)
kale, roughly chopped	3/4 cup (50g)
roughly chopped parsley	1 tablespoon
buckwheat	1/4 cup (40g)

Serves 1

INSTRUCTIONS

1. In a small saucepan, heat oil over low to moderate heat and cook the onion, garlic, carrot, celery, chili (if used) and herbs carefully till the onion becomes soft but not golden brown.

2. Stir in the tomatoes, stock, and puréed tomatoes and bring to a simmer. Add the beans and allow to cook for thirty minutes.

3. Add the kale and prepared food for the next five to ten minutes, then introduce the parsley.

4. In the meantime, as per the box directions, fry the buckwheat, drain, and serving with the stew.

STRAWBERRY BUCKWHEAT TABBOULEH

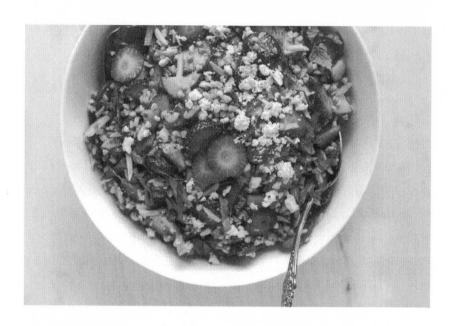

Ingredients	Quantity
buckwheat	1/3 cup (50g)
ground turmeric	1 tablespoon
avocado	1/2 cup (80g)
tomato	3/8 cup (65g)
red onion	1/8 cup (20g)
Medjool dates, pitted	1/8 cup (25g)
capers	1 tablespoon
parsley	3/4 cup (30g)
strawberries, hulled	2/3 cup (100g)
extra-virgin olive oil	1 tablespoon

juice of lemon	½
arugula	1-ounce (30g)

Serves 1

INSTRUCTIONS

1. Make the buckwheat with the turmeric as indicated on the box. Chill and set it aside.

2. Start cutting the avocado, basil, red onion, capers, dates, and parsley thinly and blend with the fresh buckwheat. Get the strawberries and blend oil and lemon juice gently in a dish. Serve on an earthenware platter.

MISO-MARINATED BAKED COD WITH STIR-FRIED GREENS AND SESAME

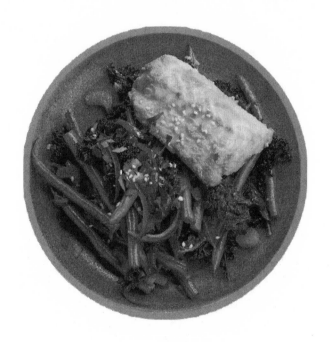

Ingredients	Quantity
Miso	3 1/2 teaspoons (20g)
Mirin	1 tablespoon
extra-virgin olive oil	1 tablespoon
skinless cod fillet	1 x 7-ounce (200g)
red onion, sliced	1/8 cup (20g)
celery, sliced	3/8 cup (40g)
garlic cloves, finely sliced	2

Thai chili, finely sliced	1
finely sliced fresh ginger	1 teaspoon
green beans	3/8 cup (60g)
kale, roughly chopped	3/4 cup (50g)
sesame seeds	1 teaspoon
parsley, roughly chopped	2 tablespoons (5g)
tamari (or soy sauce if you are not avoiding gluten)	1 tablespoon
buckwheat	1/4 cup (40g)
ground turmeric	1 teaspoon

Serves 1

INSTRUCTIONS

1. Blend the oil with the mirin and 1 teaspoon miso. Massage the cod all over and marinate for thirty minutes.
2. Heat the oven to 220 ° C (4250F).
3. Cook the cod for ten minutes.
4. In the meantime, heat the residual oil in a large skillet or wok. Stir-fry the onion for a few minutes, then add the celery, chili, garlic, ginger, green beans, and kale. Mix and roast till the kale is crispy. To help the frying process you might have to add a little water to the skillet.
5. Fry the buckwheat along with the turmeric as per the manufacturer's instructions.
6. Stir-fry the parsley, sesame seeds, and tamari and present with the buckwheat and salmon.

SOBA (BUCKWHEAT NOODLES) IN A MISO BROTH WITH TOFU, CELERY, AND KALE

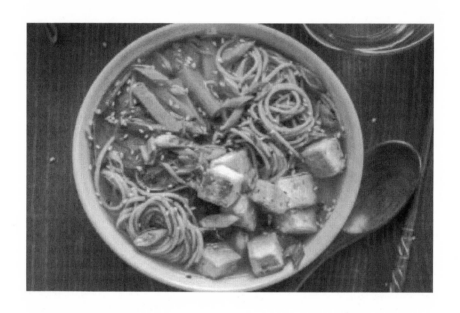

Ingredients	Quantity
soba (buckwheat noodles)	3 ounces (75g)
extra-virgin olive oil	1 tablespoon
red onion, sliced	1/8 cup (20g)
garlic cloves, finely sliced	2
finely sliced fresh ginger	1 teaspoon
vegetable stock, plus a little extra, if necessary	1 1/4 cups (300ml)
miso paste	1 3/4 tablespoons (30g)
kale, roughly chopped	3/4 cup (50g)

celery, roughly chopped	1/2 cup (50g)
sesame seeds	1 teaspoon
rm tofu, cut into ¼ - to ½ - inch (0.5 to 1cm) cubes (about 3/8 cup)	3 ½ ounces (100g)
tamari (optional; or soy sauce if not avoiding gluten)	1 teaspoon

Serves 1

INSTRUCTIONS

1. Put the noodles in a saucepan filled with hot water and cook for five to eight minutes or as indicated on the box.

2. In a frying pan, start adding the oil, then the garlic, onions, ginger, and fry in the oil over a moderate flame until tender, but not golden brown. Stir in stock and miso and bring to a simmer.

3. Add the kale and celery to the miso broth and cook slowly for five minutes (try not to heat the miso as you demolish the taste and make its texture smudgy). As needed, add a little more stock.

4. Add the fried noodles and sesame seeds and let the tofu heat up. Serve in a bowl slathered with some tamari.

SIRT SUPER SALAD

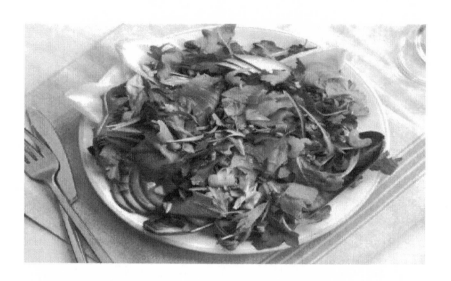

Ingredients	Quantity
arugula	1 3/4 ounces (50g)
endive leaves	1 3/4 ounces (50g)
smoked salmon slices	3 1/2 ounces (100g)
avocado, peeled, stoned, and sliced	1/2 cup (80g)
celery including leaves, sliced	1/2 cup (50g)
red onion, sliced	1/8 cup (20g)
walnuts, chopped	1/8 cups (15g)
capers	1 tablespoon

large Medjool date, pitted and chopped	1
extra-virgin olive oil	1 tablespoon
juice of lemon	¼
parsley, chopped	1/4 cup (10g)

Serves 1

INSTRUCTIONS

1. Position the salad leaf on a tray or in a plastic bucket. Blend the rest of the ingredients and place over the foliage.

VARIATIONS

1. Substitute the roasted salmon with 11/3 cups (100 g) canned green lentils or grilled Le Puy lentils for a **lentil** sirt super salad.
2. Replace the roasted salmon with a chopped cooked chicken breast, for a fantastic **chicken** sirt salad.
3. Replace the roasted salmon with canned tuna for a **tuna** sirt super salad (in oil or water, as preferred).

CHAR-GRILLED BEEF WITH A RED WINE JUS, ONION RINGS, GARLIC KALE, AND HERB-ROASTED POTATOES

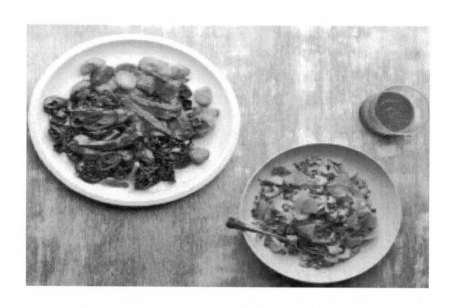

Ingredients	Quantity
potatoes, peeled and cut into	1/2 cup (100g)
diced pieces	3/4-inch (2cm)
extra-virgin olive oil	1 tablespoon
parsley, finely sliced	2 tablespoons (5g)
red onion, sliced into rings	1/3 cup (50g)
kale, sliced	2 ounces (50g)
garlic cloves, finely sliced	2

beef tenderloin (about 1 ½ inches or 3.5cm thick) or sirloin steak (¾ inch or 2cm thick)	1 x 4- to 5-ounce (120 to 150g)
red wine	3 tablespoons (40ml)
beef stock	5/8 cup (150ml)
tomato purée	1 teaspoon
corn flour, dissolved in 1 tablespoon water	1 teaspoon

Serves 1

INSTRUCTIONS

1. Heat the oven to 425°F (220°C). Put the potatoes in hot water and bring them to a simmer for four to five minutes, then strain and wash. Put one teaspoon of oil in a large skillet and cook the potatoes for thirty-five to forty minutes in the preheated oven. Flip the potatoes every ten minutes to make sure the frying is even. Remove from the heat and when finished, top with the minced garlic and stir well.

2. Cook the onion over a moderate flame in one teaspoon of oil for approximately five minutes, until smooth and crispy. Keep warm.

3. Heat the kale for two to three minutes, then strain. In ½ teaspoon of oil, cook the garlic slowly for one minute, till thin but not gray. Insert the kale and cook for another one to two minutes till soft. Keep warm.

4. Warm up an ovenproof frying pan at a high temperature. Coat the meat with ½ teaspoon of oil and roast over moderate to high heat in the skillet, depending on how you like your meat (see our baking time guide). If you like your meat medium, it would be best to caramelize it and then move it to an oven set at 425oF (220oC) for the specified time.

5. Take the meat from the saucepan and let it rest. Add remaining meat remaining and wine to the skillet. Reduce the wine by cooking for a highly concentrated flavor.

6. Add the dry ingredients and tomato purée to the skillet and bring to a simmer, then introduce the corn flour paste to thicken till the required consistency is reached. Add any of steak juices and serving with the fried potatoes, kale, onion rings, and wine sauce.

STEAK COOKING TIMES

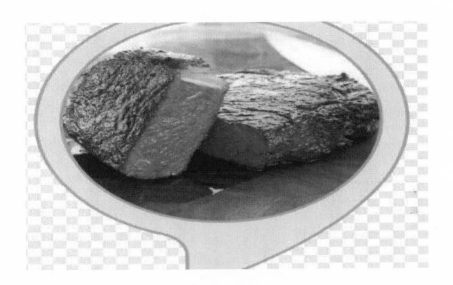

Ingredients	Quantity
TENDERLOIN	1$^{1/2}$-INCH-THICK (3.5CM)
Blue	about 1 $^{1/2}$ minutes each side
Rare	about 2 $^{1/4}$ minutes each side
Medium-rare	about 3 $^{1/4}$ minutes each side
Medium	about 4 $^{1/2}$ minutes each side
SIRLOIN STEAK	**3/4-INCH-THICK (2CM)**
Blue	about 1 minute each side
Rare	about 1 $^{1/2}$ minutes each side
Medium-rare	about 2 minutes each side
Medium	about 2 $^{1/4}$ minutes each side

KIDNEY BEAN MOLE WITH BAKED POTATO

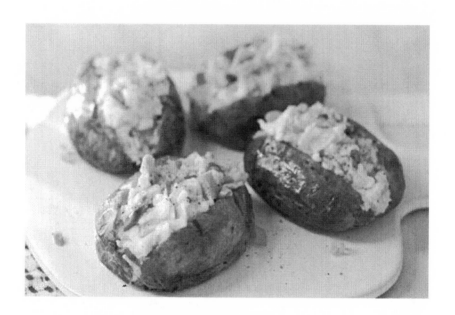

Ingredients	Quantity
red onion, finely sliced	1/4 cup (40g)
finely sliced fresh ginger	1 teaspoon
garlic cloves, finely sliced	2
Thai chili, finely sliced	1
teaspoon extra virgin olive oil	1
ground turmeric	1 teaspoon
ground cumin	1 teaspoon
ground clove	pinch of

ground cinnamon	pinch of
medium baking potato	1
canned chopped tomatoes	7/8 cup (190g)
brown sugar	1 teaspoon
red bell pepper, cored, seeds removed, and roughly chopped	1/3 cup (50g)
vegetable stock	5/8 cup (150ml)
cocoa powder	1 tablespoon
sesame seeds	1 teaspoon
peanut butter (smooth if available, but chunky is best)	2 teaspoons
canned kidney beans	7/8 cup (150g)
parsley, chopped	2 tablespoons (5g)

Serves 1

INSTRUCTIONS

1. Heat the oven to 400°F (200°C).
2. In a small saucepan, cook the onion, garlic, ginger, and chili in oil over a moderate flame for about ten minutes until soft. Add the ingredients and continue cooking for one to two more minutes.

3. Put the potato on a cookie sheet and roast until caramelized (largely dependent on how caramelized you like it) for forty-five to fifty minutes.

4. In the meantime, add to the casserole the sugar, tomatoes, red pepper, stock, peanut butter, cocoa powder, sesame seeds, and kidney beans and cook slowly for forty-five to sixty minutes.

5. At the end, adorn with parsley. Slice the potato in half and serve covered in mole.

SIRTFOOD OMELET

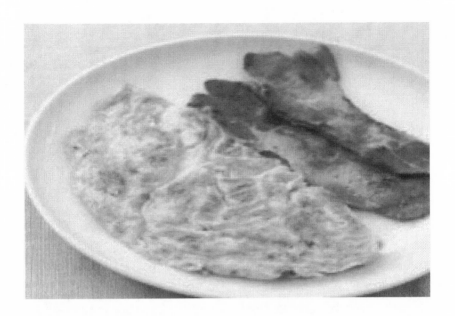

Ingredients	Quantity
sliced streaky bacon (or 2 rashers, smoked or regular, depending on your taste)	about 2 ounces (50g)
medium eggs	3
red endive, thinly sliced	1 1/4 ounces (35g)
parsley, finely sliced	2 tablespoons (5g)
Turmeric	1 teaspoon
extra virgin olive oil	1 teaspoon

Serves 1

INSTRUCTIONS

1. Spray a deep fryer with a nonstick cooking spray. Chop the bacon into small slices and cook until crispy over a high temperature. You shouldn't need to add oil the bacon contains sufficient fat for cooking. Remove from heat and drain on a paper towel to remove grease.

2. Beat the eggs and blend in the endive, the parsley and the turmeric. Cut the bacon into squares and mix in the eggs.

3. Warm oil in the pan, warm but not smoking. Add the egg mixture and scramble it with a spatula. Rotate the pan to make an even omelet. Decrease the heat and cook it bit more. Trace the spatula around the corners and under the eggs and flip the omelet before serving.

BAKED CHICKEN BREAST WITH WALNUT AND PARSLEY PESTO AND RED ONION SALAD

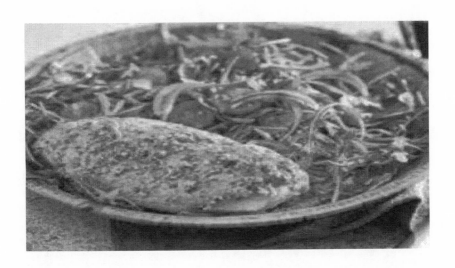

Ingredients	Quantity
parsley	3/8 cup (15g)
walnuts	1/8 cup (15g)
Parmesan cheese, grated	4 teaspoons (15g)
extra-virgin olive oil	1 tablespoon
juice of lemon	½
water	3 tablespoons (50ml)
skinless chicken breast	5 ½ ounces (150g)
red onions, finely sliced	1/8 cup (20g)
red wine vinegar	1 teaspoon
arugula	1 ¼ ounces (35g)

cherry tomatoes, cut in half	2/3 cup (100g)
balsamic vinegar	1 teaspoon

Serves 1

INSTRUCTIONS

1. To prepare the pesto, put the parsley, parmesan, walnuts, olive oil, a little of the lemon juice, and some water in a skillet or blender and mix unless a smooth paste. Progressively add more water to have the quality you want.

2. In the refrigerator, caramelize the roast chicken with one tablespoon of pesto and the residual lemon juice for thirty minutes, or longer as needed.

3. Preheat the oven to 400°F (200°C).

4. Warm an ovenproof deep fryer over moderate to high heat. In the marinade, roast the chicken for one minute, then move the saucepan to the oven to bake for eight minutes or till roasted.

5. Caramelize the onions for five to ten minutes in red wine vinegar and drain.

6. After roasting, remove the chicken from the heat, spoon another tablespoon of pesto over it, and then let the chicken's warmth dissolve the pesto. Wrap in foil and set aside for five min to rest before serving.

7. Mix the balsamic vinegar with the tomatoes, arugula, and onion. Add to the meat and cover with leftover pesto.

WALDORF SALAD

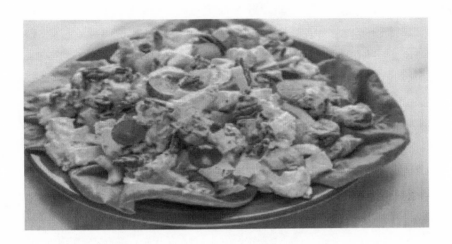

Ingredients	Quantity
celery including leaves, roughly chopped	1 cup (100g)
apple, roughly chopped	1/2 cup (50g)
walnuts, roughly chopped	3/8 cup (50g)
red onion, roughly chopped	1 tablespoon (10g)
parsley, chopped	2 tablespoons (5g)
capers	1 tablespoon
extra-virgin olive oil	1 tablespoon
balsamic vinegar	1 teaspoon
juice of lemon	¼
Dijon mustard	1/4 teaspoon
arugula	about 2 ounces (50g)
endive leaves	about 1 ¹/² ounces (35g)

Serves 1

INSTRUCTIONS

1. Mix the parsley and capers, the celery including the foliage, onion, walnuts, and apple.
2. To prepare the dressing: whisk the vinegar, oil, lemon juice, and mustard in a bottle or bowl.
3. Serve with the celery mixture on top of the endive and arugula as a coating.

ROASTED EGGPLANT WEDGES WITH WALNUT AND PARSLEY PESTO AND TOMATO SALAD

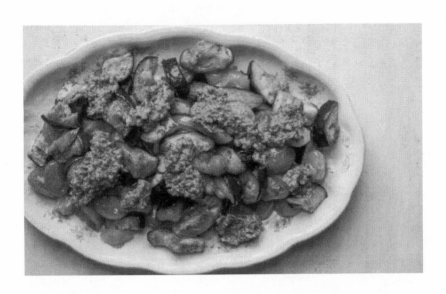

Ingredients	Quantity
parsley	1/2 cup (20g)
walnuts	3/4 ounces (20g)
Parmesan cheese (or use a vegetarian or vegan alternative), grated	1/8 cup (20g)
extra-virgin olive oil	1 tablespoon
juice of lemon	¼
water	3 tablespoons (50ml)

eggplant, quartered	1 small (around $5^{1/2}$ ounces or 150g)
red onions, sliced	1/8 cup (20g)
red wine vinegar	1 teaspoon (5ml)
arugula	1 1/4 ounces (35g)
cherry tomatoes	2/3 cup (100g)
balsamic vinegar	1 teaspoon (5ml)
Serves 1	

INSTRUCTIONS

1. Heat the oven to 400°F (200°C).
2. Put the parsley, walnuts, Parmesan, olive oil and s quarter of the lemon juice in a bowl or mixer to make the pesto with a fine consistency. Progressively add the water till you have a good consistency — dense enough for the eggplant to adhere to.
3. Cover the eggplant with some pesto and reserve the remainder for serving. Put on a cookie sheet and grill for twenty-five to thirty minutes till the gray, smooth, and soggy eggplant is golden.
4. In the meantime, coat the red onion with red wine vinegar and set aside — this should smooth and caramelize the onion. Drain off the vinegar and serve.
5. Mix the arugula, tomatoes, and drained onion and sprinkle the salad with balsamic vinegar. Serve with soft eggplant, covered with the leftover pesto.

SIRTFOOD SMOOTHIE

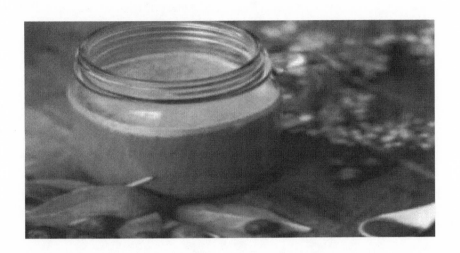

Ingredients	Quantity
plain Greek yogurt (or vegan alternative, such as soy or coconut yogurt)	3/8 cup (100g)
walnut halves	6
strawberries, hulled	8 to 10 medium size
handful of kale, stalks removed	
dark chocolate (85 percent cocoa solids)	3/4 ounce (20g)
Medjool date, pitted	1
ground turmeric	1/2 teaspoon
thin sliver of Thai chili	(1 to 2mm)
unsweetened almond milk	7/8 cup (200ml)

Serves 1

INSTRUCTIONS

1. In a food processor, rumble ingredients until buoyant and light.

STUFFED WHOLEWHEAT PITA

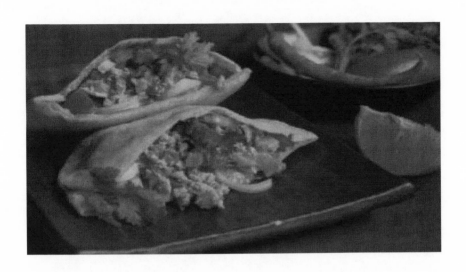

Ingredients	Quantity
FOR A MEAT OPTION	
cooked turkey slices, chopped	3 ounces (80g)
cheddar cheese, diced	3/4-ounce (20g)
cucumber, diced	1/4 cup (35g)
red onion, chopped	1/4 cup (35g)
arugula, chopped	1-ounce (25g)
walnuts, roughly chopped	1 1/2 to 2 tablespoons (10 to 15g)
FOR THE DRESSING	
extra-virgin olive oil	1 tablespoon
balsamic vinegar	1 tablespoon

dash of lemon juice

FOR A VEGAN OPTION

hummus	2 to 3 tablespoons
cucumber, diced	1/4 cup (35g)
red onion, chopped	1/4 cup (35g)
1-ounce (25g) arugula, chopped	to taste
walnuts, roughly chopped	1 1/2 to 2 tablespoons (10 to 15g)

FOR THE VEGAN DRESSING

extra-virgin olive oil	1 tablespoon
dash of lemon juice	to taste

Serves 1

INSTRUCTIONS

1. Entire wheat pitas are a good way to add a lot of sirtfoods into a quick lunch or versatile filling meal. You can carry it and get innovative with the amount, but inevitably all you do is pile on the additives and it's good to go.

BUTTERNUT SQUASH AND DATE TAGINE WITH BUCKWHEAT

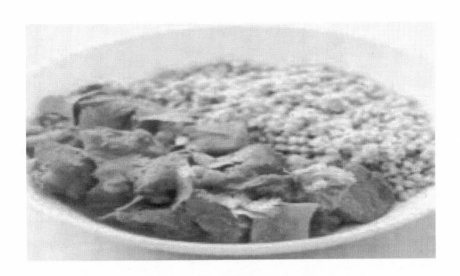

Ingredients	Quantity
extra virgin olive oil	3 teaspoons
red onion, finely sliced	1
finely sliced fresh ginger	1 tablespoon
garlic cloves, finely sliced	4
Thai chilies, finely sliced	2
ground cumin	1 tablespoon
cinnamon stick	1
ground turmeric	2 tablespoons
chopped tomatoes	2 x 14-ounce cans (400g each)

vegetable stock	1 1/4 cups (300ml)
Medjool dates, pitted and chopped	2/3 cup (100g)
of chickpeas, drained and rinsed	1 x 14-ounce can (400g)
butternut squash, peeled and cut into bite-size pieces	2 1/2 cups (500g)
buckwheat	1 1/4 cups (200g)
fresh coriander, chopped	2 tablespoons (5g)
fresh parsley, chopped	1/4 cup (10g)

Serves 4

INSTRUCTIONS

1. Heat the oven to 400°F (200°C).
2. Use 2 teaspoons of oil to cook the onion, garlic, ginger, and chili for two or three minutes. Add the cumin and cinnamon and 1 teaspoon of turmeric; then bake one to two minutes longer.
3. Start adding the tomatoes, stock, dates, and chickpeas and slowly boil for 45-60 minutes. You may need to insert a little more water to get a thick, sticky uniformity and ensure that skillet doesn't get dry.
4. Put the squash in a saucepan, mix with the residual oil and grill until crispy and roasted for thirty minutes.

5. Towards the end of the cooking process, make the tagine and frying the buckwheat with a spoonful of turmeric as per manufacturer guidelines.

6. Add the grilled squash, coriander and parsley to the tagine and serve with the buckwheat.

BUTTER BEAN AND MISO DIP WITH CELERY STICKS AND OATCAKES

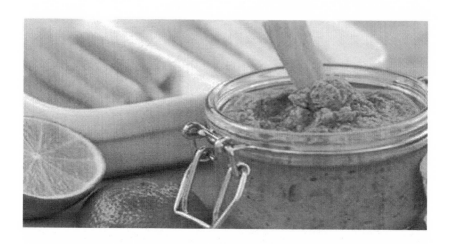

Ingredients	Quantity
of butter beans, drained and rinsed	2 x 14-ounce cans (400g each)
extra virgin olive oil	3 tablespoons
brown miso paste	2 tablespoons
juice and grated zest of 1/2 unwaxed lemon	to taste
medium scallions, trimmed and finely sliced	4
garlic clove, squeezed	1
Thai chili, finely sliced	1/4
celery sticks, to serve	to taste
oatcakes, to serve	to

Serves 4

INSTRUCTIONS

1. Put the first 7 components into blender, reaching a rough consistency.
2. Serve the celery sticks with the oatcakes as a sauce.

YOGURT WITH MIXED BERRIES, CHOPPED WALNUTS, AND DARK CHOCOLATE

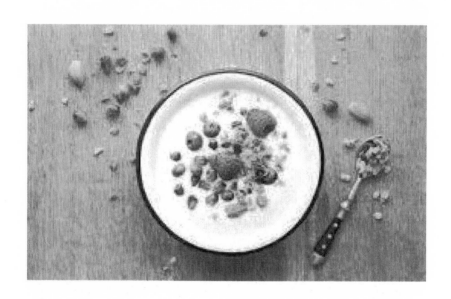

Ingredients	Quantity
mixed berries	about 1 1/3 cups (125g)
plain Greek yogurt (or vegan alternative, such as soy or coconut yogurt)	2/3 cup (150g)
walnuts, chopped	1/4 cup (25g)
dark chocolate (85 percent cocoa solids), grated	1 1/2 tablespoons (10g)

Serves 1

INSTRUCTIONS

1. Add your favorite berries to a bowl and cover with the yogurt.
2. Sprinkle with the dark chocolate and walnuts.

CHICKEN AND KALE CURRY
WITH BOMBAY POTATOES

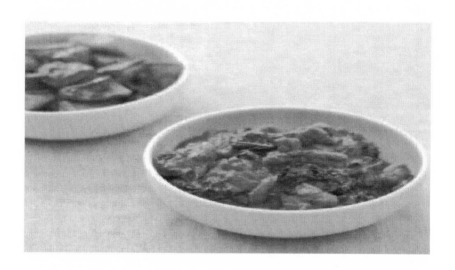

Ingredients	Quantity
skinless, boneless chicken breasts, cut into bite-size pieces	4 x 4 ½ - to 5 ½ -ounce (120 to 150g)
extra virgin olive oil	4 tablespoons
ground turmeric	3 tablespoons
red onions, sliced	2
Thai chilies, finely sliced	2
garlic cloves, finely sliced	3
finely sliced fresh ginger	1 tablespoon
mild curry powder	1 tablespoon
can chopped tomatoes	1 x 14-ounce (400g)

chicken stock	2 1/8 cups (500ml)
coconut milk	7/8 cup (200ml)
cardamom pods	2
cinnamon stick	1
russet potatoes	1 1/3 pounds (600g)
parsley, chopped	1/4 cup (10g)
kale, chopped	2 2/3 cups (175g)
coriander, chopped	2 tablespoons (5g)

Serves 4

INSTRUCTIONS

1. Massage the chicken breast in one teaspoon of oil and one tablespoon of turmeric and marinate for thirty minutes.

2. Roast the meat over a high temperature (the meat should fry well with the adequate oil in the marinade) for four to five minutes just until golden brown. Remove from heat and aside.

3. Heat 1 spoonful of oil in the roasting pan over moderate heat and add the onion, chili, garlic, and ginger. Roast for about ten minutes till soft, then introduce the curry powder and another turmeric spoonful; cook for one to two minutes.

4. Add the tomatoes to the pan and roast for another two minutes. Include stock, coconut milk, cardamom and cinnamon stick and boil for forty-five to sixty minutes. Inspect the pan frequently to make sure it doesn't dry up — you may need more oil.

5. Heat the oven to 425 ° F (220 ° C). Prepare the potatoes while your gravy is cooking. Scrub and slice into small pieces. Put the residual teaspoon of turmeric in the boiling water and simmer for five minutes.

6. Drain well and let dry steam for ten minutes. Potatoes will be white and waxy.

7. Move to a baking dish, mix in the residual oil and grill till nicely browned and crunchy for 30 minutes. (Throw the parsley away before eating.)

8. Add kale, roasted chicken, and coriander when the sauce is to taste, and cook for another five minutes to make sure the meat is cooked through. Serve with the potatoes.

SPICED SCRAMBLED EGGS

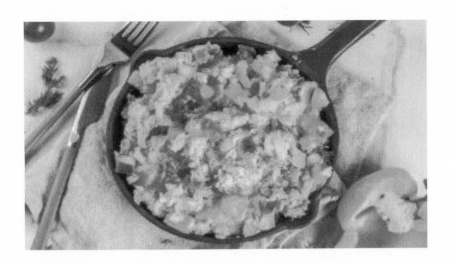

Ingredients	Quantity
extra virgin olive oil	1 teaspoon
red onion, finely sliced	1/8 cup (20g)
Thai chili, finely sliced	1/2
medium eggs	3
milk	1/4 cup (50ml)
ground turmeric	1 teaspoon
parsley, finely sliced	2 tablespoons (5g)

Serves 1

INSTRUCTIONS

1. In a skillet, heat the oil and fry the red onion and chili till smooth but not brown.

2. Blend the eggs, milk, turmeric, and oil. Add to the skillet and cook for a few minutes over low to moderate heat. Scramble the beaten eggs continuously and stir to avoid burning. Serving at the texture desired. Some like their eggs soft.

SIRT CHILI CON CARNE

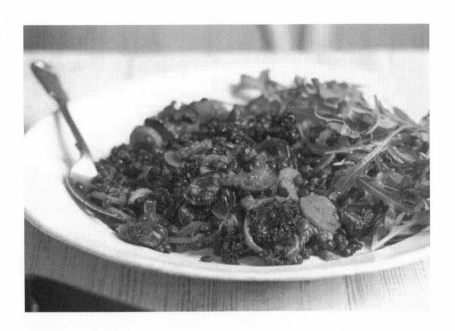

Ingredients	Quantity
red onion, finely sliced	1
garlic cloves, finely sliced	3
Thai chilies, finely sliced	2
extra-virgin olive oil	1 tablespoon
ground cumin	1 tablespoon
ground turmeric	1 tablespoon
lean ground beef (5 percent fat)	1 pound (450g)
red wine	5/8 cup (150ml)

red bell pepper, cored, seeds removed and cut into bite-size pieces	1
cans chopped tomatoes	2 x 14-ounce (400g)
tomato purée	1 tablespoon
cocoa powder	1 tablespoon
canned kidney beans	7/8 cup (150g)
beef stock	1 1/4 cups (300ml)
fresh coriander, chopped	2 tablespoons (5g)
fresh parsley, chopped	2 tablespoons (5g)
buckwheat	1 cup (160g)

Serves 4

INSTRUCTIONS

1. Sauté the garlic, onion, and chili in the oil for two or three minutes over moderate heat in a large frying pan, then add the other ingredients and continue cooking for a minute or two.

2. Add the chopped beef and cook over a medium-high temperature for two or three minutes till the meat golden brown. Add the red wine let steam to reduce by half.

3. Add the red pepper, tomatoes, puréed tomatoes, cocoa, kidney beans and boil for one hour. Occasionally, add a little more water but keep a thick, sticky uniformity.

4. Stir in the spices right before eating.

5. In the meantime, as per the manufacturer's directions, fry the buckwheat and serve with the chili.

MUSHROOM AND TOFU SCRAMBLE

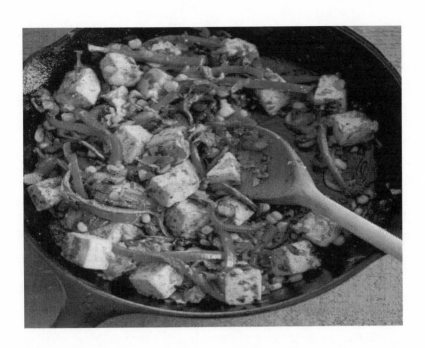

Ingredients	Quantity
extra-rm tofu	3 1/2 ounces (100g)
ground turmeric	1 teaspoon
mild curry powder	1 teaspoon
kale, roughly chopped	1/3 cup (20g)
extra virgin olive oil	1 teaspoon
red onion, thinly sliced	1/8 cup (20g)
Thai chili, thinly sliced	1/2
mushrooms, thinly sliced	3/4 cup (50g)
parsley, finely sliced	2 tablespoons (5g)

Serves 1

INSTRUCTIONS

1. Roll tofu in paper towel to drain.

2. Blend the curry and turmeric powder, then add water till a light pulp is formed. Heat the kale for two to three minutes.

3. Warm the oil over medium-high heat in a pan and roast the onion, chili, and mushrooms for two or three minutes before browning and softening begins.

4. Cut the tofu into small bites and transfer to the saucepan. Cover with the seasoning mixture and completely blend. Fry for two or three minutes over moderate heat so the ingredients are roasted through and the tofu begins browning.

5. Add the kale and cook for a minute over a moderate flame. Add the parsley, blend well, and serve.

SMOKED SALMON PASTA WITH CHILI AND ARUGULA

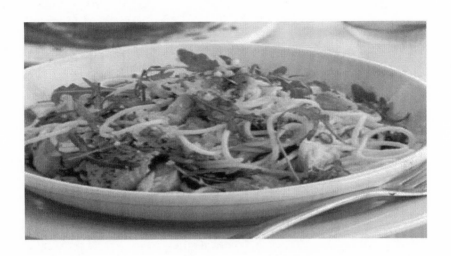

Ingredients	Quantity
extra virgin olive oil	2 tablespoons
red onion, finely sliced	1
garlic cloves, finely sliced	2
Thai chilies, finely sliced	2
cherry tomatoes, cut in half	1 cup (150g)
white wine	1/2 cup (100ml)
buckwheat pasta	9 to 11 ounces (250 to 300g)
smoked salmon	9 ounces (250g)
capers	2 tablespoons
juice of lemon	½
arugula	2 ounces (60g)
parsley, chopped	1/4 cup (10g)

Serves 4

INSTRUCTIONS

1. In a broiler pan, heat one teaspoon of the oil over a moderate flame. Stir in the onion, garlic, chili, and fry till smooth but not dark brown.

2. Add the tomatoes and bake for one or two minutes. To reduce by half, simmer the white wine.

3. Prepare the pasta in boiling water with one tablespoon of oil for eight to ten minutes based texture, then drain.

4. Split the salmon into pieces and add the capers, lemon juice, arugula, parsley, and tomato into the saucepan. Mix in the sauce, blend, and eat. Sprinkle oil over top to taste.

BUCKWHEAT PASTA SALAD

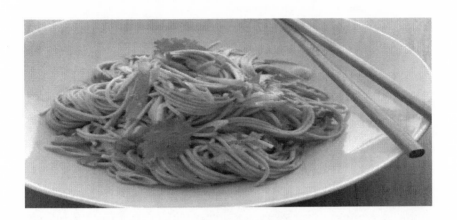

Ingredients	Quantity
buckwheat pasta, cooked according to the package instructions	2 ounces (50g)
handful of arugula	large
handful of basil leaves	small
cherry tomatoes, cut in half	8
avocado, diced	1/2
olives	10
extra-virgin olive oil	1 tablespoon
pine nuts	2 1/2 tablespoons (20g)

Serves 1

INSTRUCTIONS

1. Incorporate all the spices, except for the pine nuts, and organize them on a tray, with the nuts over the top.

BUCKWHEAT PANCAKES WITH STRAWBERRIES, DARK CHOCOLATE SAUCE, AND SQUEEZED WALNUTS

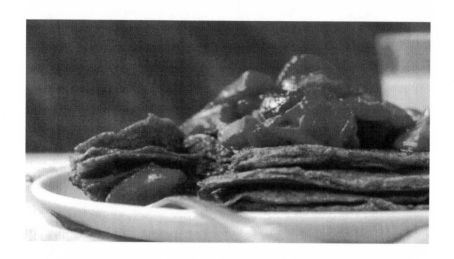

Ingredients	Quantity
FOR THE PANCAKES	
milk	1 1/2 cups (350ml)
buckwheat our	7/8 cup (150g)
large egg	1
extra-virgin olive oil, for cooking	1 tablespoon
FOR THE CHOCOLATE SAUCE	
dark chocolate (85 percent cocoa solids)	3 1/2 ounces (100g)

milk	1/3 cup (85ml)
double cream	1 tablespoon
extra-virgin olive oil	1 tablespoon
TO SERVE	
strawberries, hulled and chopped	2 cups (400g)
walnuts, chopped	7/8 cup (100g)

Makes 6 to 8, depending on size

INSTRUCTIONS

1. Add all ingredients besides the olive oil to a food processor to start the pancake mix with a smooth texture. It must not be too dense or too runny. (Any leftover mixture can be kept in an enclosed jar or in the refrigerator for up to five days. Make sure to blend properly before using again.)

2. Melt the dark chocolate in a heat-proof bowl over a tray of boiling water to melt the chocolate sauce. When warmed, blend well with the milk, and whisk vigorously. Then add the double cream and olive oil. By keeping the water in the oven, you can maintain the sauce hot, boiling gently till your pancakes are prepared.

3. Microwave a frying pan till it begins smoking, then add the olive oil to begin making the pancakes.

4. Place some of the mixture in the middle of the bowl, then move the excess mixture around till you've coated the entire surface. You might need to apply a little more of the mixture to do this. If your saucepan is hot enough, you would just need to cook the pancakes on each side for a minute or so.

5. Use a spatula to remove the pancake from the bottom of the pan, after it is brown on top, then flip over. Avoid splitting in pieces. Fry the other side for a moment and move to a plate or tray.

6. Garnish with strawberries and arrange upwards. Proceed with more pancakes, as desired.

7. Across each pancake, drizzle a decent amount of sauce and scatter sliced walnuts.

8. If at first your pancakes are too thick or tough adjust the formula and you refine your method. Ultimately, you'll become an expert.

TOFU AND SHIITAKE MUSHROOM SOUP

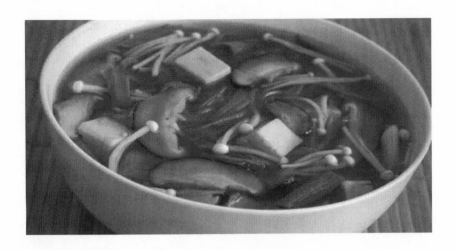

Ingredients	Quantity
dried wakame (seaweed)	1/3 ounce (10g)
vegetable stock	1-quart (1 liter)
shiitake mushrooms, sliced	7 ounces (200g)
miso paste	1/3 cup (120g)
block rm tofu, cut into small cubes	1 x 14-ounce (400g)
scallions, trimmed and sliced on the diagonal	2
Thai chili, finely sliced (optional)	1

Serves 4

INSTRUCTIONS

1. Drench the wakame for ten minutes in hot water then rinse. Add the stock and bring to a simmer, then introduce the mushrooms and gently boil for 1-2 minutes.

2. Thin the miso paste with some of the hot stock in a pan to completely dissolve. Add the miso and tofu to the remaining ingredients, being careful not to let the soup simmer too long as it will ruin the delicate taste. When serving, add the soaked wakame, scallions, and chili.

SIRTFOOD BITES

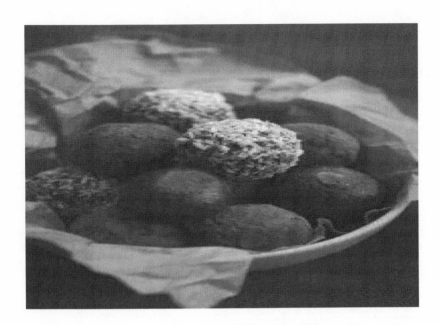

Ingredients	Quantity
walnuts	1 cup (120g)
dark chocolate (85 percent cocoa solids), broken into cocoa nibs	1 ounce (30g) pieces; or 1/4 cup
Medjool dates, pitted	9 ounces (250g)
cocoa powder	1 tablespoon
ground turmeric	1 tablespoon
extra-virgin olive oil	1 tablespoon
the scraped seeds OR vanilla extract	1 vanilla pod OR 1 teaspoon

water   1 to 2 tablespoons

Makes 15 to 20 bites

INSTRUCTIONS

1. Put the walnuts and dark chocolate in a food processor and pulse till the powder is perfect.

2. Add the rest of the ingredients apart from the water and blend until the mixtures has turned into a ball. You might not have to add water if you don't want it too thin.

3. Form the ball into bite-size pellets using your hand and cool in an enclosed jar for at least one hour until time to eat. With more chocolate or dry coconut, roll to change the texture, if you prefer. Store it in your refrigerator for up to one week.

QUINOA, CHICKPEA AND TURMERIC CURRY

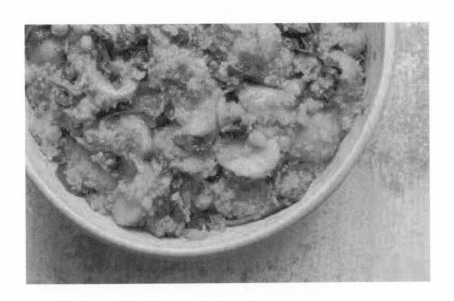

Ingredients	Quantity
new potatoes, cut in half	500g
garlic cloves, squeeze	3
ground turmeric	3 teaspoons
ground coriander	1 teaspoon
chilli flakes or (powder)	1 teaspoon
ground ginger	1 teaspoon
chopped tomatoes	400g
coconut milk	400g
tomato purée	1 tablespoon

pepper and salt	To taste
quinoa	180g
chickpeas, drained and rinsed	400g
spinach	150g
Serves 6	

INSTRUCTIONS

1. Put the potatoes in a pan with cool water and then steam for around 25 minutes so a knife can easily enter. Drain well.

2. In a large saucepan containing the potatoes, add the garlic, turmeric, coriander, chili, ginger, coconut milk, tomato purée and tomatoes. Bring to a simmer, season with pepper and salt, then add 300ml of boiling water into the quinoa.

3. Decrease heat, cover and continue cooking. Mix every five minutes, or so, for a total of thirty minutes to ensure nothing sticks. (This takes a long time to prepare, but the same as preparing quinoa in all additives.)

4. Midway through frying, add the chickpeas. When five minutes are remaining, add the spinach and stir before it wilts. Once the quinoa is fluffy and crunchy, it's done.

5. If you want a touch of heat, apply a sliced red chili at the same time as all the other peppers to the frying curry.

SAVORY TURMERIC PANCAKES WITH LEMON YOGURT SAUCE

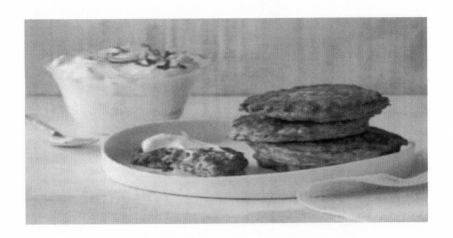

for the pancakes

Ingredients	Quantity
ground turmeric	2 teaspoons
ground cumin	1½ teaspoons
salt	1 teaspoon
ground coriander	1 teaspoon
garlic powder	½ teaspoon
ground black pepper	½ teaspoon freshly
head broccoli, cut into florets	1
large eggs, lightly beaten	3
plain unsweetened almond milk	2 tablespoons

almond flour	1 cup
coconut oil	4 teaspoons

Serves 8 pancakes

For The Yogurt Sauce

Ingredients	Quantity
Greek yogurt	1 cup plain
garlic clove, minced	1
lemon juice (from 1 lemon), to taste	1 to 2 tablespoons
ground turmeric	¼ teaspoon
mint leaves (fresh), minced	10
lemon zest (from 1 lemon)	2 teaspoons

INSTRUCTIONS

1. To make the yogurt sauce: In a bowl, mix the yogurt, garlic, lemon juice, turmeric, mint, and zest. To taste, spice with citrus juice. Set aside or put it in the fridge until ready to eat.

2. To make the pancakes: Blend the turmeric, cumin, salt, coriander, garlic, and pepper in a shallow pot.

3. Put the broccoli in a blender. Blend into tiny chunks until the florets are minced. Move the broccoli to a large mixing bowl, then add in the eggs, almond milk, and almond flour. Add the spice mixture and mix well.

4. Heat 1 teaspoon of coconut oil over medium to low heat in a nonstick frying pan. Pour 1⁄4 of the batter into the pan.

5. Heat the pancake until you see tiny bubbles on the top, and the base is light brown, for 2 to 3 minutes.

6. Flip over and cook the pancake for another 2 to 3 minutes. Transmit the baked pancakes to an oven-safe dish and put them in a 200 ° F oven to keep warm.

7. Making the 3 remaining pancakes, with the residual oil and batter.

BLUEBERRY SMOOTHIE

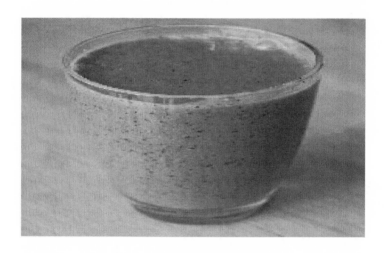

Ingredients	Quantity
ripe banana	1
blueberries	100g
blackberries	100g
natural yogurt	2 tablespoons
milk	200ml
calories	**160**
Ready in	**2 minutes**
Serves 2	

INSTRUCTIONS

This yogurt smoothie has a rich, creamy taste.

1. Mix all of ingredients until all light and fluffy.

BLUEBERRY BANANA PANCAKES WITH CHUNKY APPLE COMPOTE AND GOLDEN TURMERIC LATTE

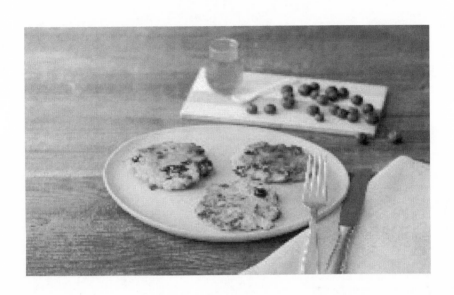

Blueberry Banana Pancakes

Ingredients	Quantity
bananas	6
eggs	6
rolled oats	150g
baking powder	2 teaspoons
salt	¼ teaspoon
blueberries	25g

Chunky Apple Compote

Ingredients	Quantity
apples	2
dates (pitted)	5
lemon juice	1 tablespoon
cinnamon powder	1/4 teaspoon
pinch salt	To taste

Golden Turmeric Latte

Ingredients	Quantity
coconut milk	3 cups
turmeric powder	1 teaspoon
cinnamon powder	1 teaspoon
raw honey	1 teaspoon
black pepper (increases absorption)	Pinch
ginger root (fresh and peeled)	Tiny piece
cayenne pepper (optional)	Pinch

INSTRUCTIONS

For the Blueberry banana pancakes:

1. In a high-speed blender, place the rolled oats and process for 1 minute or until oat flour develops. Tip:

ensure your processor is really dry or else the mixture get watery!

2. Add the bananas, eggs, baking powder and salt to the mixer and pulse two minutes to form a smooth batter.

3. Carefully place the blueberries in a large mixing bowl with the batter.

4. Allow the baking powder to sit for 10 minutes until activated.

5. Add a dollop of butter to a skillet over medium-high heat (this will make them very fluffy and crispy!). Insert spoonful's of the blueberry pancake mix and fry on each side until perfectly golden.

For the chunky apple compote

1. Core and rough chop the apples.

2. Place in a food processor with 2 spoonful's of water and a pinch of salt. Pulse your chunky apple compote to desired texture.

For the Golden Turmeric Latte

1. In a high-speed mixer, combine all ingredients till smooth.

2. Cook over moderate flame in a small saucepan for 4 minutes until hot but not boiling.

3. Enjoy!

BUCKWHEAT SUPERFOOD MUESLI

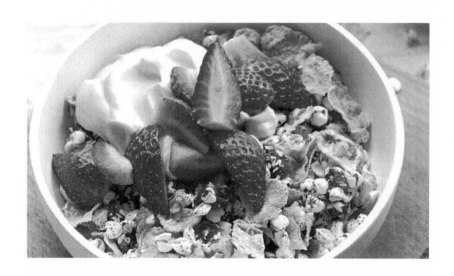

Ingredients	Quantity
buckwheat flakes	20g
buckwheat puffs	10g
desiccated coconut or coconut flakes	15g
Medjool dates (pitted and chopped)	40g
walnuts, finely sliced	15g
cocoa nibs	10g
strawberries (chopped and hulled)	100g

plain Greek yogurt OR vegan alternative like (soy or coconut yogurt)	100g

INSTRUCTIONS

1. Mix the above-mentioned ingredients together, leaving out the strawberries and yogurt if not to be eaten immediately.

NOTE

Mix the remaining ingredients and place them in an airtight jar if you'd like to make it in quantity and even cook it the night before. The next day all you have to do is mix the strawberries and yogurt and it's good to go.

MOCHA CHOCOLATE MOUSSE

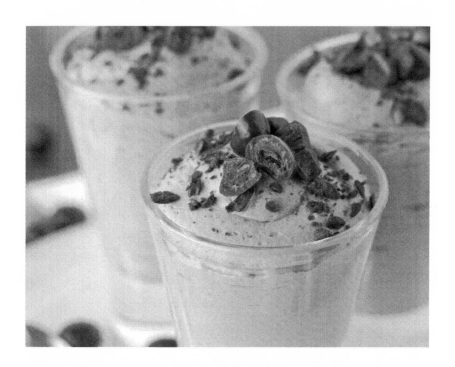

Everybody appreciates chocolate mousse and this one has a beautiful airy texture. It's fast and easy to make, and best served the day after.

Ingredients	Quantity
dark chocolate (cocoa solids 85%)	250g
medium free-range eggs (separated)	6
strong black coffee	4 tablespoons

almond milk	4 tablespoons
chocolate coffee beans	to decorate

Serves 4–6

INSTRUCTIONS

1. Melt the chocolate in a bowl of softly boiling water in a water bath, ensuring the surfaces are not in contact. Turn off the heat and remove the bowl.

2. Allow the molten chocolate to cool at room temperature.

3. When the melting chocolate has achieved the ambient temperature, swirl in the egg yolks one at a time then add in the coffee and almond milk.

4. Stir the egg whites with a manual or electric mixer until sharp peaks form, then add a few heaping spoonful's to the chocolate mixture to soften it.

5. Add the remainder and gently stir with a big spoon.

6. Pour the mousse to individual serving glasses and smooth the top as desired

7. Let stand at least 2 hours, preferably overnight, using plastic wrap, then chill.

8. Adorn with chocolate coffee beans.

RAW BROWNIE BITES

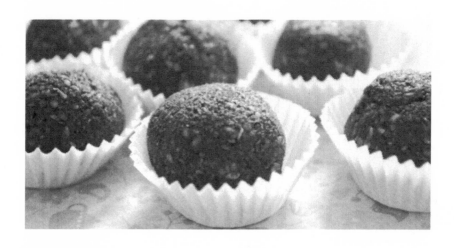

Ingredients	Quantity
whole walnuts	2½ cups
almonds	¼ cup
Medjool dates	2½ cups
cacao powder	1 cup
vanilla extract	1 teaspoon
sea salt	⅛ - ¼ teaspoon
Ready in	**5 minutes**

Serves 6

INSTRUCTIONS

1. Put everything in a mixing bowl till well blended.
2. Form into bites and arrange on a cookie sheet and refrigerate for thirty minutes to two hours.

MOROCCAN SPICED EGGS

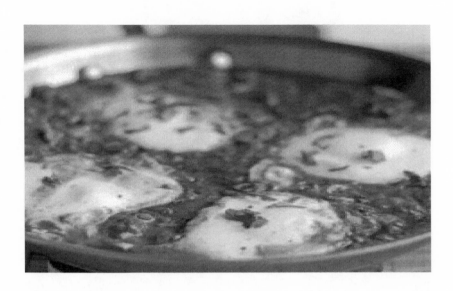

Ingredients	Quantity
olive oil	1 teaspoon
shallot (finely sliced and peeled)	1
red (bell) pepper, (deseeded and finely sliced)	1
garlic clove, (peeled and finely sliced)	1
courgette (zucchini), (peeled and finely sliced)	1
tomato puree (paste)	1 tablespoon
mild chili powder	½ teaspoon

ground cinnamon	¼ teaspoon
ground cumin	¼ teaspoon
salt	½ teaspoon
chopped tomatoes	1 × 400g (14oz)
chickpeas in water	1 x 400g (14oz)
flat-leaf parsley (small handful)	10g (1/3oz)
medium eggs	4 at room temperature
Calories	**394**
Ready in	**50 MINUTES**

Serves 2

INSTRUCTIONS

1. In a frying pan, heat the oil, insert the shallots and red (bell) pepper and cook slowly for five minutes. Stir in the garlic and courgette (zucchini) and cook for a few minutes.

2. Add the tomato puree (paste), salt and spices and mix.

3. Add the sliced tomatoes and chickpeas (soaked in liquor) and keep on a moderate heat. Boil the sauce for thirty minutes uncovered. It will bubble softly and decrease by around one-third in volume.

4. Take the sliced parsley off the heat and stir well.

5. Set the microwave temperature to 200C/180C fan/350F.

6. Take the tomato sauce to a moderate boiling point when you are ready to cook the eggs, then switch to a clean, oven-proof bowl.

7. Crack the eggs and slowly drop them into the stew. Wrap the bowl in foil, then bake for 10-15 minutes.

8. Serving the delicious concoction with the eggs on top in small cups.

VIETNAMESE TURMERIC FISH WITH HERBS & MANGO SAUCE

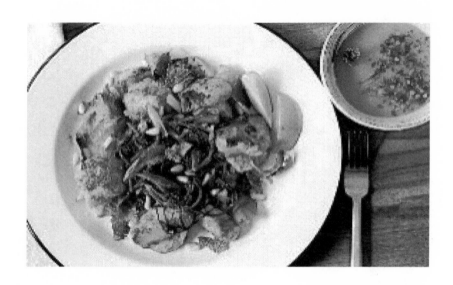

Fish

Ingredients	Quantity
fresh cod fish (skinless and boneless), cut it ½ inch thick and about 2-inch piece wide	1 ¼ lbs.
coconut oil in pan and fry the fish	2 tablespoons (plus a few more tablespoon if necessary)
sea salt to taste	pinch

Fish marinade

Ingredients	Quantity
turmeric powder	1 tablespoon
sea salt	1 teaspoon
Chinese cooking wine OR dry sherry	1 tablespoon
minced ginger	2 teaspoons
olive oil	2 tablespoons
Marinate for at least 1 hr.	

Infused Scallion and Dill Oil

Ingredients	Quantity
scallions (slice into long thin shape)	2 cups
fresh dill	2 cups of
sea salt to taste	pinch

Mango dipping sauce

Ingredients	Quantity
medium sized ripe mango	1
rice vinegar	2 tablespoons
Juice of lime	1/2
garlic clove	1
dry red chili pepper (stir in before serving)	1 teaspoon

Toppings

Fresh cilantro	to taste
Lime juice	to taste
Nuts (pine nuts or cashew)	to taste

Preparation time: 15 mins Cook time 30 mins Total 45 minutes.

Serves: 4

INSTRUCTIONS

1. Marinate the fish for one hour or overnight.
2. Add all ingredients in a mixing bowl for Mango Dipping Sauce and combine until texture is obtained.

To pan-fry the fish:

1. Heat 2 tablespoons of coconut oil on a high temperature in a large, nonstick skillet. Add the marinated fish when hot. Note: put the fish slices in separately segregated into two or more quantities if needed.
2. A loud sizzle will be heard, after which you can reduce the heat.
3. Do not turn or relocate the fish until after about 5 minutes, you see a golden-brown skin.

4. Sprinkle with a tablespoon of sea salt. If required, add more coconut oil.

5. When the fish is in golden brown, flip it gently to the other side. Transfer to a large plate when done. Note: the saucepan should have some residual oil left to suffuse with scallions and dill.

To make the scallion and dill Infused oil:

1. Heat the residual oil over medium to high heat in a frying pan, add 2 cups of scallions and 2 cups of dill.

2. Stir about fifteen seconds, till the scallions and dill simmer.

3. Season with a sprinkle of sea salt.

4. Place the scallion and dill infused oil over the fish and garnish with fresh cilantro, lime, and nuts and mango sauce.

SIRTFOOD DIET'S SHAKSHUKA

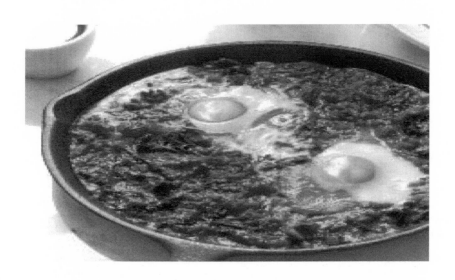

Ingredients	Quantity
Extra virgin olive oil	1 teaspoon
Red onion, finely sliced	40g
Garlic clove, finely sliced	1
Celery, finely sliced	30g
Bird's eye chili, finely sliced	1
Ground cumin	1 teaspoon
Ground turmeric	1 teaspoon
Paprika	1 teaspoon
Tinned chopped tomatoes	400g
Kale, stems removed, finely sliced	30g

Chopped parsley	1 tablespoon
Medium eggs	2
Ready in	**40 minutes**
Serves 1	

INSTRUCTIONS

1. Cook tomatoes over medium to low heat a small deep saucepan. Add the oil and brown the onion, garlic, celery, chili, and spices for approximately one minute.

2. Remove the tomatoes and let the sauce to boil slowly, stirring regularly for twenty minutes.

3. Add the kale and continue cooking for another five minutes. If the sauce is too thick, just add a bit of water.

4. Mix in the parsley for a rich flavor.

5. Make tiny wells in the sauce, then break an egg into each of them.

6. With the heat very low, cover and cook ten to twelve minutes.

7. The whites will be firm while the yolks are still soft.

8. Reheat for an extra three to four minutes if you like well-done yolks.

9. Serve right away directly from the pan.

SIRTFOOD DIET'S BRAISED PUY LENTILS

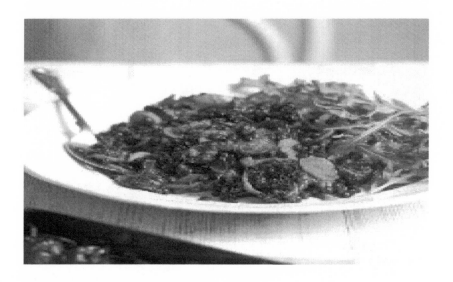

Ingredients	Quantity
cherry tomatoes, cut in half	8
extra virgin olive oil	2 teaspoons
red onion (thinly sliced)	40 g
garlic clove, finely sliced	1
celery (thinly sliced)	40 g
carrots (thinly sliced and peeled)	40 g
paprika	1 teaspoon
thyme (fresh or dry)	1 teaspoon
puy lentils	75 g
vegetable stock	220 ml

kale, finely sliced	50 g
parsley, finely sliced	1 tablespoon
Rocket	20 g
Preparation time	40 – 50 minutes

Serves: 1

INSTRUCTIONS

1. Heat the oven to 120°C/gas ½.
2. Place the tomatoes in a small metal pan and roast for thirty-five to forty minutes in the oven.
3. Prepare and cook the stock over low – moderate heat. Add a tablespoon of olive oil with red onion, garlic, celery, and carrot and cook for one to two minutes.
4. Stir in the thyme then the paprika, and simmer for another minute.
5. Wash the lentils in a sieve and add them to the stock.
6. Bring to a simmer, then increase heat and slowly boil covered for twenty minutes.
7. Stir after about seven minutes, adding some water if the level is reduced.
8. Stir in the kale and continue to cook mixture for another ten minutes.

9. Mix in the parsley and roasted tomatoes when the lentils are baked.

10. Top with a teaspoon of olive oil sprinkle over with rocket (arugula).

SALMON SIRT SUPER SALAD

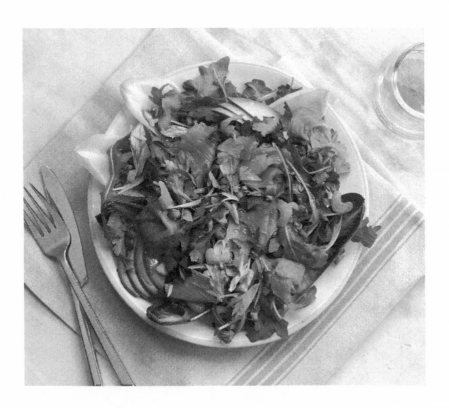

Ingredients	Quantity
rocket	50g
chicory leaves	50g
smoked salmon slices (alt. cooked chicken breast, lentils, or tinned tuna)	100g
avocado (stoned, sliced and peeled)	80g

celery (sliced)	40g
red onion (sliced)	20g
walnuts, finely sliced	15g
capers	1 tbs
large Medjool date (chopped and pitted)	1
extra-virgin olive oil	1 tbs
Juice of lemon	¼
parsley, finely sliced	10g
celery leaves or lovage, finely sliced	10g

INSTRUCTIONS

1. Organize the salad leave on a nice serving dish.
2. Blend the rest of the ingredients and arrange over the leaves.

CHINESE-STYLE PORK WITH PAK CHOI

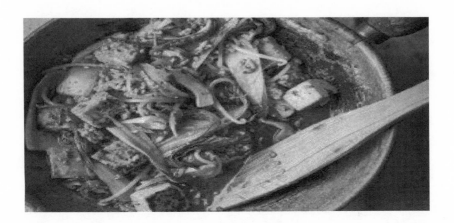

Ingredients	Quantity
firm tofu (cut into large cubes)	400g
corn flour	1 tablespoon
Water	1 tablespoon
chicken stock	125ml
rice wine	1 tablespoon
tomato puree	1 tablespoon
brown sugar	1 teaspoon
soy sauce	1 tablespoon
clove garlic (squeezed and peeled)	1
fresh ginger (grated and peeled)	1 thumb (5cm)

rapeseed oil	1 tablespoon
shiitake mushrooms (sliced)	100g
shallot (sliced and peeled)	1
choi sum or pak choi (cut into thin slices)	200g, 400g (10% fat)
beansprouts	100g
large handful parsley, finely sliced	(20g)
CALORIES	**377**

Serves: 4

INSTRUCTIONS

1. Put the tofu on a paper towel from the fridge. Set aside.
2. Blend the corn flour and water in a small bowl and remove all the lumps.
3. Stir into the poultry stock the rice wine, tomato purée, brown sugar, and soy sauce. Add the smashed garlic and ginger, then stir.
4. Heat the oil to a temperature in a wok or large deep fryer.
5. Add the shiitake mushrooms and stir-fry until glossy for two to three minutes.
6. Remove the mushrooms from the skillet and set aside using a slotted spoon to drain.

7. Add the tofu to the saucepan and stir-fry until golden on all sides. Cover and set aside.

8. Add the shallots and pak choi to the wok, stir-fry for two minutes.

9. Fry until heated through, then add the sauce, decrease the heat a bit, and let the sauce to steam for a couple of minutes with the meat.

10. Add the beansprouts, mushrooms, and tofu to the saucepan and cook.

11. Turn off heat, mix in some parsley and serve hot.

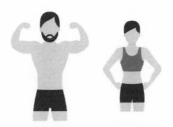

Chapter 8:
Maintain a healthy life

DOING EXERCISE WITH THE DIET

The Sirtfood Diet is all about eating those foods designed to promote sustained weight loss and well-being by nature. Even with the advantages you see from adopting the diet, you might slip into the pitfall of eschewing exercise. This is endorsed by many diet books that say how ineffective exercise is compared with following the right weight loss diet. And it is right, we can't exercise with a bad diet. It's not what has been intended to drive weight loss. It is expensive and there are too many frontiers to cross.

So, it's true that until we see stars or perform an Olympian's feats, there's no need to pound the treadmill — but what about general everyday movement?

The truth is we are now much less involved than we used to be. The age of technology has ensured that physical activity is practically factored out of our everyday lives with all the changes made. We don't really have to bother with the whole business of being active unless we actually want to. We can roll out of bed, drive to work, take the elevator, sit at a desk the whole day, drive home, eat and watch TV before rolling back into bed. Then do the same the next day and the next.

Whatever sport or physical activity you enjoy is appropriate. Pleasure and exercise do not have to be mutually exclusive! And their social aspect enriches team or community events even more. It's also about everyday things like taking the bike instead of the car, or getting off the bus one stop earlier, or just parking farther away to increase the distance you've got to walk. Take the stairs and not the elevator. Go outside and garden. Play in the park with your family or go out with the dog. Everything counts. Anything that has you up and going will activate your sirtuin genes frequently and at moderate strength, maximizing the benefits of the Sirtfood Diet.

Engaging in physical activity while eating a diet rich in sirtfood gives you the biggest bang for the sirtfood buck.

SIRTFOOD DIET DURING PREGNANCY

The Sirtfood Diet isn't recommended for women trying to conceive, or if you're pregnant or nursing. It is a powerful diet for weight loss however. Don't be put off eating plenty of sirtfoods on their own, as these are exceptionally healthy foods to be included as part of a balanced and varied pregnancy diet.

SIRTFOOD DIET FOR CHILDREN

The Sirtfood diet is not intended for children. This doesn't mean that children will miss out on the excellent health benefits provided by having more sirtfoods in their overall diet. A large majority of extremely healthy foods will help them attain a balanced or nutritious diet. Many of the recipes planned for the stage 2 diet were produced with families in mind, including children's taste buds. The likes of the sirtfood pizza, the chili con carne and the sirtfood bites are perfect child-friendly foods with a higher nutritional value than their usual food offerings.

Although most sirtfoods are extremely healthy for children to eat, the green juice, which is too concentrated in fat burning sirtfoods, is not recommended. We also advise against caffeine sources, such as coffee and green tea.

SIRTFOOD DIET FOR PEOPLE ON MEDICATION

The Sirtfood Diet is perfect for many people, but it can alter the course of certain diseases and the drug recommended by your doctor due to its powerful effects on fat burning and wellbeing.

Similarly, other medications are not ideal while in a fasting condition.

During the Sirtfood Diet trial, each individual's suitability was assessed before they embarked on the diet, particularly those taking medication. Obviously, we can't do that for you, so if you're suffering from a major health problem, taking prescribed medicines or have other reasons to worry about, go slowly if at all.

CANCER PREVENTION FOODS

All cancer and nutrition studies point to eating plant-based foods for their phytonutrients and other special compounds. Target five to nine regular fruit and vegetables of all kinds — especially these six megastars.

Broccoli

All brassica vegetables (think cauliflower, cabbage, kale) have cancer-fighting ingredients, but broccoli is the only one without a hefty portion of sulforaphane, a highly potent component that increases the body's preventive enzymes and washes out chemicals that can cause cancer.

Helps fight breast, liver, lung, prostate, skin, stomach, and bladder cancers.

Your Rx: The more broccoli, the better so research suggests. Include it wherever you can from salads and omelets to the top of a pizza.

Berries

All berries are packed with micronutrients that battle cancer. But black raspberries in particular contain high quantities of phytochemicals called anthocyanins, which slow the progression of premalignant cells and prevent new blood cells from establishing and potentially feeding a cancerous tumor.

Helps fight colon, esophageal, oral, and skin cancers.

Your Rx: Half a cup of berries a day can improve your health.

Tomatoes

This juicy fruit is the major diet source of lycopene, a carotenoid that delivers the red hue to tomatoes. And that's great news because in a research study in Nutrition and Cancer, lycopene was found to stop endometrial cancer cell growth. Endometrial cancer kills close to 8,000 people a year.

Helps fight endometrial, lung, prostate, and stomach cancers.

Your Rx: The greatest advantage comes from roasted tomatoes (think pasta sauce!), as the heat treatment increases the level of lycopene your body can absorb.

Walnuts

Their phytosterols (cholesterol-like molecules found in plants) have been shown to limit estrogen neurons in breast cancer cells, potentially slowing the growth of these cells.

Helps fight breast and prostate cancers

Your Rx: Having 1 ounce of walnuts per day deliver the best advantages.

Garlic

Phytochemicals in garlic have been found to stop nitrosamine formation and carcinogens in the stomach (and in the intestines under certain conditions) when you ingest nitrates, a commonly consumed preservative, according to Béliveau. In fact, Iowa Women's Health researchers showed that women with the highest quantities of garlic in their diets had a 50 percent lower risk of colon cancer than those who ate the least amount.

Helps fight breast, colon, esophageal, and stomach cancers

Your Rx: Cut a fresh, crushed garlic clove (crushing helps release beneficial enzymes) and add to tomato sauce (which is rich in lycopene) while simmering.

Beans

Research performed by Michigan State University found that black and navy beans considerably reduced the incidence of colon cancer in rats, partly because a diet rich in legumes continues to increase fatty acid butyrate levels, which have beneficial effects against cancer growth in high concentrations. The research found that canned beans were especially helpful in preventing breast cancer in rats, as published in the paper Crop Science.

Helps fight breast and colon cancers

Your Rx: Eat a serving of legumes a few days per week (from either a can or dry beans washed and roasted) to your daily green or other vegetable routine.

What not to eat: animal fats

While scientists are still trying to find out which foods get the most cancer-preventing benefits, we know what not to eat if you'd like to keep yourself safe.

Animal fats: Meat, cheese, and butter may be rich in saturated fat that has been linked to obesity — a large predictor of cancer. Opt for leaner sources of protein like fish, low-fat dairy, and those good-for-you beans.

What not to eat: processed meats

A ballpark hot dog or a couple of slices of bacon will not kill you once in a while, but just don't make them a mainstay of your diet. Many steaks have high number of nitrites and nitrates, preservatives that potentially increase your risk of significant quantities of gastrointestinal and other cancers.

What not to drink: excessive alcohol

Hold on after one drink! Too much tippling is linked to an increased risk of mouth, esophagus, and breast cancers.